Bacterial Diseases

Edited by

Muhammad Imran Qadir

Institute of Molecular Biology & Biotechnology
Bahauddin Zakariya University, Multan
Pakistan

Bacterial Diseases

Editor: Muhammad Imran Qadir

ISBN (Online): 978-981-14-7376-0

ISBN (Print): 978-981-14-7374-6

ISBN (Paperback): 978-981-14-7375-3

© 2020, Bentham Books imprint.

Published by Bentham Science Publishers Pte. Ltd. Singapore. All Rights Reserved.

BENTHAM SCIENCE PUBLISHERS LTD.
End User License Agreement (for non-institutional, personal use)

This is an agreement between you and Bentham Science Publishers Ltd. Please read this License Agreement carefully before using the ebook/echapter/ejournal (**"Work"**). Your use of the Work constitutes your agreement to the terms and conditions set forth in this License Agreement. If you do not agree to these terms and conditions then you should not use the Work.

Bentham Science Publishers agrees to grant you a non-exclusive, non-transferable limited license to use the Work subject to and in accordance with the following terms and conditions. This License Agreement is for non-library, personal use only. For a library / institutional / multi user license in respect of the Work, please contact: permission@benthamscience.net.

Usage Rules:

1. All rights reserved: The Work is the subject of copyright and Bentham Science Publishers either owns the Work (and the copyright in it) or is licensed to distribute the Work. You shall not copy, reproduce, modify, remove, delete, augment, add to, publish, transmit, sell, resell, create derivative works from, or in any way exploit the Work or make the Work available for others to do any of the same, in any form or by any means, in whole or in part, in each case without the prior written permission of Bentham Science Publishers, unless stated otherwise in this License Agreement.
2. You may download a copy of the Work on one occasion to one personal computer (including tablet, laptop, desktop, or other such devices). You may make one back-up copy of the Work to avoid losing it.
3. The unauthorised use or distribution of copyrighted or other proprietary content is illegal and could subject you to liability for substantial money damages. You will be liable for any damage resulting from your misuse of the Work or any violation of this License Agreement, including any infringement by you of copyrights or proprietary rights.

Disclaimer:

Bentham Science Publishers does not guarantee that the information in the Work is error-free, or warrant that it will meet your requirements or that access to the Work will be uninterrupted or error-free. The Work is provided "as is" without warranty of any kind, either express or implied or statutory, including, without limitation, implied warranties of merchantability and fitness for a particular purpose. The entire risk as to the results and performance of the Work is assumed by you. No responsibility is assumed by Bentham Science Publishers, its staff, editors and/or authors for any injury and/or damage to persons or property as a matter of products liability, negligence or otherwise, or from any use or operation of any methods, products instruction, advertisements or ideas contained in the Work.

Limitation of Liability:

In no event will Bentham Science Publishers, its staff, editors and/or authors, be liable for any damages, including, without limitation, special, incidental and/or consequential damages and/or damages for lost data and/or profits arising out of (whether directly or indirectly) the use or inability to use the Work. The entire liability of Bentham Science Publishers shall be limited to the amount actually paid by you for the Work.

General:

1. Any dispute or claim arising out of or in connection with this License Agreement or the Work (including non-contractual disputes or claims) will be governed by and construed in accordance with the laws of Singapore. Each party agrees that the courts of the state of Singapore shall have exclusive jurisdiction to settle any dispute or claim arising out of or in connection with this License Agreement or the Work (including non-contractual disputes or claims).
2. Your rights under this License Agreement will automatically terminate without notice and without the

need for a court order if at any point you breach any terms of this License Agreement. In no event will any delay or failure by Bentham Science Publishers in enforcing your compliance with this License Agreement constitute a waiver of any of its rights.

3. You acknowledge that you have read this License Agreement, and agree to be bound by its terms and conditions. To the extent that any other terms and conditions presented on any website of Bentham Science Publishers conflict with, or are inconsistent with, the terms and conditions set out in this License Agreement, you acknowledge that the terms and conditions set out in this License Agreement shall prevail.

Bentham Science Publishers Pte. Ltd.
80 Robinson Road #02-00
Singapore 068898
Singapore
Email: subscriptions@benthamscience.net

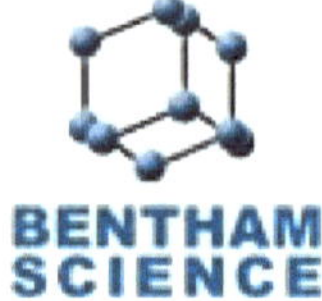

CONTENTS

PREFACE

The book contains topics on Bacterial Diseases like Anthrax, pneumonia, Bacterial Tooth Decay, Bubonic plague, Tuberculosis, Leptospirosis, Syphilis, Leprosy, Burn Infection, Gas gangrene, Spontaneous bacterial peritonitis, Relapsing fever, Rat-bite fever, Brucellosis and many more. Each disease has been explained by its symptoms, diagnosis, causes, and treatment. At the start, there is a summary of the whole chapter, so that one can easily take the concept within the limited time. Keywords are also included for a quick indicator of the chapter. The book contains introductory material for pharmacy, medical, & dental students, also M Phil, Ph.D. for Pharmacology, Botany, Zoology, Microbiology, Pharmacy, Biotechnology, and all other related health sciences subjects. It is also very helpful for common people.

As an editor and author, and on the behalf of my co-authors, I declare that we have no conflict of interests, neither financial nor any other. Moreover, nothing to acknowledge.

Muhammad Imran Qadir
Institute of Molecular Biology & Biotechnology
Bahauddin Zakariya University, Multan
Pakistan

List of Contributors

Afshan Saleem — Institute of Molecular Biology & Biotechnology, Bahauddin Zakariya University, Multan, Pakistan

Adeela Awan — Institute of Molecular Biology & Biotechnology, Bahauddin Zakariya University, Multan, Pakistan

Asma Jan Muhammad — Institute of Molecular Biology & Biotechnology, Bahauddin Zakariya University, Multan, Pakistan

Azra Yasmeen — Institute of Molecular Biology & Biotechnology, Bahauddin Zakariya University, Multan, Pakistan

Aleena Ahmad Somroo — Institute of Molecular Biology & Biotechnology, Bahauddin Zakariya University, Multan, Pakistan

Afia Javaid — Institute of Molecular Biology & Biotechnology, Bahauddin Zakariya University, Multan, Pakistan

Ayesha Altaf — Institute of Molecular Biology & Biotechnology, Bahauddin Zakariya University, Multan, Pakistan

Basra Manzoor — Institute of Molecular Biology & Biotechnology, Bahauddin Zakariya University, Multan, Pakistan

Fatima Rehan — Institute of Molecular Biology & Biotechnology, Bahauddin Zakariya University, Multan, Pakistan

Fahad Zafar — Institute of Molecular Biology & Biotechnology, Bahauddin Zakariya University, Multan, Pakistan

Ghalia Batool Alvi — Institute of Molecular Biology & Biotechnology, Bahauddin Zakariya University, Multan, Pakistan

Hafiza Sobia Khan — Institute of Molecular Biology & Biotechnology, Bahauddin Zakariya University, Multan, Pakistan

Hira Jamil — Institute of Molecular Biology & Biotechnology, Bahauddin Zakariya University, Multan, Pakistan

Iqra Shahzadi — Institute of Molecular Biology & Biotechnology, Bahauddin Zakariya University, Multan, Pakistan

Iqra Jamshaid — Institute of Molecular Biology & Biotechnology, Bahauddin Zakariya University, Multan, Pakistan

Irtiqa Masood — Institute of Molecular Biology & Biotechnology, Bahauddin Zakariya University, Multan, Pakistan

Iqra Ali Yameen — Institute of Molecular Biology & Biotechnology, Bahauddin Zakariya University, Multan, Pakistan

Jaleel Ahmad — Institute of Molecular Biology & Biotechnology, Bahauddin Zakariya University, Multan, Pakistan

Muhammad Imran Qadir — Institute of Molecular Biology & Biotechnology, Bahauddin Zakariya University, Multan, Pakistan

Muhammad Mubashar Idrees — Institute of Molecular Biology & Biotechnology, Bahauddin Zakariya University, Multan, Pakistan

Mahreen Fatima	Institute of Molecular Biology & Biotechnology, Bahauddin Zakariya University, Multan, Pakistan
Mahnoor Khan	Institute of Molecular Biology & Biotechnology, Bahauddin Zakariya University, Multan, Pakistan
Munaza Gilani	Institute of Molecular Biology & Biotechnology, Bahauddin Zakariya University, Multan, Pakistan
Maria Rizvi	Institute of Molecular Biology & Biotechnology, Bahauddin Zakariya University, Multan, Pakistan
Maleeha Batool	Institute of Molecular Biology & Biotechnology, Bahauddin Zakariya University, Multan, Pakistan
Momal Tariq Tariq	Institute of Molecular Biology & Biotechnology, Bahauddin Zakariya University, Multan, Pakistan
Nadia Wazir	Institute of Molecular Biology & Biotechnology, Bahauddin Zakariya University, Multan, Pakistan
Rabia Hussain	Institute of Molecular Biology & Biotechnology, Bahauddin Zakariya University, Multan, Pakistan
Rimsha Khan	Institute of Molecular Biology & Biotechnology, Bahauddin Zakariya University, Multan, Pakistan
Rameen Fatima	Institute of Molecular Biology & Biotechnology, Bahauddin Zakariya University, Multan, Pakistan
Rahat Bano	Institute of Molecular Biology & Biotechnology, Bahauddin Zakariya University, Multan, Pakistan
Ramsha Shahzad	Institute of Molecular Biology & Biotechnology, Bahauddin Zakariya University, Multan, Pakistan
Sadia Ishfaq	Institute of Molecular Biology & Biotechnology, Bahauddin Zakariya University, Multan, Pakistan
Sidra Zafar	Institute of Molecular Biology & Biotechnology, Bahauddin Zakariya University, Multan, Pakistan
Sadaf Noor	Institute of Molecular Biology & Biotechnology, Bahauddin Zakariya University, Multan, Pakistan
Shaiza Ali	Institute of Molecular Biology & Biotechnology, Bahauddin Zakariya University, Multan, Pakistan
Saif Ur Rehman	Institute of Molecular Biology & Biotechnology, Bahauddin Zakariya University, Multan, Pakistan
Shahpara Rehman	Institute of Molecular Biology & Biotechnology, Bahauddin Zakariya University, Multan, Pakistan
Saba Ghafoor	Institute of Molecular Biology & Biotechnology, Bahauddin Zakariya University, Multan, Pakistan
Sidra Noureen	Institute of Molecular Biology & Biotechnology, Bahauddin Zakariya University, Multan, Pakistan
Zunaira Akhtar	Institute of Molecular Biology & Biotechnology, Bahauddin Zakariya University, Multan, Pakistan

CHAPTER 1

Anthrax: A *Bacillus Anthracis* Infection

Muhammad Imran Qadir[*] and **Sidra Zafar**

Institute of Molecular Biology & Biotechnology, Bahauddin Zakariya University, Multan, Pakistan

Abstract: Anthrax is a bacterial disease and caused by the transfer of bacterial spores. *B. anthracis* is gram-positive, non-motile, and aerobic bacteria. There are 3 types of commonly caused anthrax: inhalational anthrax, cutaneous anthrax, and gastrointestinal anthrax; each with its signs and symptoms. In the old days, anthrax is diagnosed by clinical findings and by the exposure history to bacteria. In the laboratory, the Gram staining procedure, ELISA, screening, and serologic assays are used. Antimicrobial drugs are not given at once before the appearance of symptoms unless the evidence is found that the risk is present. Some antibiotics are also found to be effective against *B. anthracis* such as chloramphenicol, tetracyclines, rifampin, and other first-generation cephalosporins. Anthrax is not transmitted from one individual to another even in case of inhalational anthrax. However, standard precautions must be taken to avoid any risk.

Key Words: Anthrax, *B. anthracis*, Ciprofloxacin, Gram Staining Procedures.

INTRODUCTION

Anthrax is a bacterial disease of lungs and skin and progressive to severe ulceration caused by *B. anthracis* in humans and animals that exists as resistant spores in soil cause disease in humans and animals who have ingested or inhaled these spores. The major source of transfer of spores in humans is contact with other infected individuals for example wool, hair, the habitat of infected animals [1].

B. anthracis is gram-positive, non-motile, and aerobic bacteria. Spore-forming *B. anthracis* is large 3.0 to 10.0 μm by 1.0 to 1.5 μm. The optimum temperature for their growth is 37°C and they naturally grow in the form of colonies. In the laboratory, it grows and appears as a single organism but they are in the form of long chains. The pathogenicity of *B. anthracis* is present in two parts of plasmids, one causes the inhibition of phagocytosis by producing a polyglutamyl capsule

[*] **Corresponding author Muhammad Imran Qadir:** Institute of Molecular Biology and Biotechnology, Bahauddin Zakariya University, Multan, Pakistan; Tel: +92-61-9210071; Ext, 1920; Fax: +92-61-9210068; E-mail: mrimranqadir@hotmail.com

Muhammad Imran Qadir (Ed.)
All rights reserved-© 2020 Bentham Science Publishers

and the other helps in the production of exotoxins and have genes for it [2].

SYMPTOMS

There are 3 types of commonly caused anthrax Fig. (**1**). In the case of inhalational anthrax, the initial attack is mild and non-specific, normally the disease is not identified at this stage. The patient bears fever, chest and abdominal pain, and cough. After some days a second stage begins suddenly and acute with fever, cyanosis, and diaphoresis. Patients have swollen lymph nodes, edema of neck and chest. This stage rapidly becomes severe and can cause death within 36 hours [3].

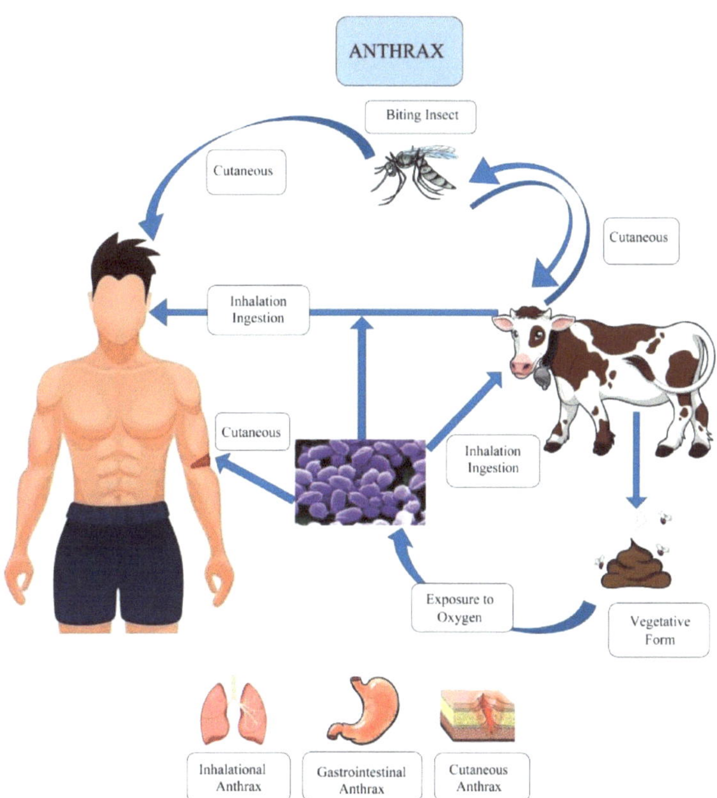

Fig. (1). Types and pathogenesis of anthrax.

In cutaneous anthrax, bacterial spores get entry into the body through wounds and cuts. After seven days of entry, primary lesions appear which are usually painless. In the next one to two days these lesions increase in size and filled with some fluid also containing leukocytes and gram-positive bacilli. Later, the lesion is enclosed by gelatinous edema. Patients have low fever and malaise. Naturally occurring anthrax is 95% of cutaneous type.

In gastrointestinal anthrax, initial symptoms start appearing after two to five days of attack consists of nausea, fever, body pains, and vomiting. These lesions are formed in caecum and ileum. In some cases, gastric ulcers are also formed.

Sometimes, inhalational anthrax may result in causing anthrax meningitis which is less common but affects the cerebrospinal fluid. Patients have 100 percent chances of death if proper antibiotics are not given [4].

DIAGNOSIS

In the old days, anthrax is diagnosed by clinical findings and by the exposure history to bacteria. With the change in the history of exposure as the spores are now transferred either by air or some other delivery means. Anthrax is identified by the general symptoms that appear on the body [5].

LABORATORY DIAGNOSIS

In the laboratory, the Gram staining procedure is used for testing either by taking a sample from lesions or blood. Tests are also performed by checking the growth that appeared on sheep's-blood agar. Different colonies appeared indicating different strains. Growth cannot be checked on MacConkey agar. Confirmatory diagnostic tests are performed by checking the growth of virulent strains on nutrient media with the little addition of carbon dioxide. Some additional confirmatory test is used which involve lysis of bacteria by gamma phage or antibody staining of the cell wall antigen.

Screening assays are also directly used by taking samples (nasal swabs). Such samples are also used to check how the infection is occurred either by inhalation or by the wound. For retrospectively purpose serologic testing is useful and samples are taken from acute phases of illness [6].

MANAGEMENT

Antimicrobial drugs are not given at once before the appearance of symptoms unless the evidence is found that the risk is present. The unnecessary use of antibiotics without the confirmation of risk is also dangerous and can cause resistance to the strain. However, prophylaxis is recommended for a long period of time. As the strains of *B. anthracis* is used for bioterrorist attack and overseas strains are resistant to certain antibiotics, only ciprofloxacin is used in initial stages [7].

Some special anthrax vaccines, containing a sterile and attenuated culture of the strain of *B. anthracis* is administrated to persons of armed forces and no side effects for the use of this drug are reported. For the effective results vaccine is given at 2 and 4 weeks and the next dose is given at 6 and 12 months. These experiments are performed on monkeys first. For the maintenance of immunity annual boosters are also given necessarily.

The supply of vaccines is very small, however, at present mostly vaccines are not recommended at first. In primates, prophylaxis treatments are given at an optimal level with the combination of some antibiotics [8].

For many decades, penicillin is being used for the treatment of anthrax and there is no resistance found in strains of bacteria for penicillin. *In vitro*, some other antibiotics are also found to be effective against *B. anthracis* such as chloramphenicol, tetracyclines, rifampin, and other first-generation cephalosporins [9].

Anthrax is not transmitted from one individual to another even in case of inhalational anthrax. However, standard precautions must be taken to avoid any risk. Patients in hospitals should be treated in separate rooms. Fluids from patients with cutaneous anthrax should not come in contact with others. Dressings of such patients are dangerous and should be wasted properly. Sporicidal solutions must be used in hospital rooms for decontamination. The public health security department should be notified immediately if there is any risk of release of *B. anthracis* [10].

CONSENT FOR PUBLICATION

Not applicable.

CONFLICT OF INTEREST

The authors declare no conflict of interest, financial or otherwise.

ACKNOWLEDGEMENTS

Declared none.

REFERENCES

[1]   Friedlander AM. Anthrax: clinical features, pathogenesis, and potential biological warfare threat. Curr Clin Top Infect Dis 2000; 20: 335-49.
[PMID: 10943532]

[2]   Vitale G, Bernardi L, Napolitani G, Mock M, Montecucco C. Susceptibility of mitogen-activated protein kinase kinase family members to proteolysis by anthrax lethal factor. Biochem J 2000; 352(Pt 3): 739-45.
[http://dx.doi.org/10.1042/bj3520739] [PMID: 11104681]

[3]   Inglesby TV, Henderson DA, Bartlett JG, *et al.* Anthrax as a biological weapon: medical and public health management. JAMA 1999; 281(18): 1735-45.
[http://dx.doi.org/10.1001/jama.281.18.1735] [PMID: 10328075]

[4]   Fish DC, Mahlandt BG, Dobbs JP, Lincoln RE. Purification and properties of *in vitro*-produced anthrax toxin components. J Bacteriol 1968; 95(3): 907-18.
[http://dx.doi.org/10.1128/JB.95.3.907-918.1968] [PMID: 4966833]

[5]   Harrison LH, Ezzell JW, Abshire TG, Kidd S, Kaufmann AF, Kaufmann AF. Evaluation of serologic tests for diagnosis of anthrax after an outbreak of cutaneous anthrax in Paraguay. J Infect Dis 1989; 160(4): 706-10.
[http://dx.doi.org/10.1093/infdis/160.4.706] [PMID: 2507648]

[6]   Belton FC, Strange RE. Studies on a protective antigen produced *in vitro* from *Bacillus anthracis:* medium and methods of production. Br J Exp Pathol 1954; 35(2): 144-52.
[PMID: 13149735]

[7]   Swartz MN. Recognition and management of anthrax--an update. N Engl J Med 2001; 345(22): 1621-6.
[http://dx.doi.org/10.1056/NEJMra012892] [PMID: 11704686]

[8]   Brachman PS, Gold H, Plotkin SA, Fekety FR, Werrin M, Ingraham NR. Field evaluation of a human anthrax vaccine. Am J Public Health Nations Health 1962; 52(4): 632-45.
[http://dx.doi.org/10.2105/AJPH.52.4.632] [PMID: 18017912]

[9]   Update: Investigation of bioterrorism-related anthrax and interim guidelines for exposure management and antimicrobial therapy, October 2001. MMWR Morb Mortal Wkly Rep 2001; 50(42): 909-19.
[PMID: 11699843]

[10]   Belton FC, Darlow HM, Henderson DW. The use of anthrax antigen to immunise man and monkey. Lancet 1956; 271(6941): 476-9.
[PMID: 13368432]

CHAPTER 2

Pneumonia: An Inflammation of Lungs

Muhammad Imran Qadir[*] and **Sadaf Noor**

Institute of Molecular Biology & Biotechnology, Bahauddin Zakariya University, Multan, Pakistan

Abstract: Inflammation of the lungs due to the attack of *Streptococcus pneumonia* bacterium is termed as pneumonia. Only one or both lungs may be affected. People of less developed countries are at substantial risk of suffering from pneumonia. Cough, high fever, breathing problems, and chest pain are some common symptoms of pneumonia. Chest X-ray, blood test, bronchoscopy are diagnostic methods to identify pneumonia. Certain antibiotics such as Penicillin, Augmentin, Erythromycin, Amoxicillin, Azithromycin, and Fluoroquinolones are used for the treatment of pneumonia. Vaccines are also available such as the pneumococcal conjugate vaccine (PCV13) and the pneumococcal polysaccharide vaccine (PPV23; Pneumovax). A healthy lifestyle including quitting smoking, hand washing, proper sleep, a healthy diet, and exercise strengthens the immune system and reduces the chances of pneumonia.

Keywords: Antibiotics, Bronchoscopy, Cough, Lungs, Pneumonia.

INTRODUCTION

Pneumonia is an inflammation of lungs due to infection caused by bacteria, viruses, or fungi. In this condition, pus accumulates in air sacs or alveoli of the lungs and blocks the air passage (Fig. **2**). Single or both lungs may be affected. *Streptococcus pneumoniae*, a gram-positive bacterium, is the most common type of bacteria which causes pneumonia [1]. *Mycoplasma pneumoniae, chlamydia pneumoniae* are some other types of bacteria that cause pneumonia [2]. According to study one million children of 5 years old or below are suffering from death due to pneumonia. 90-95% of deaths are reported to occur in less developed countries. South Asia is one of those countries which have the highest rate of deaths of children due to pneumonia [3].

[*] **Corresponding author Muhammad Imran Qadir:** Institute of Molecular Biology and Biotechnology, Bahauddin Zakariya University, Multan, Pakistan; Tel: +92-61-9210071; Ext. 1920; Fax: +92-61-9210068; E-mail: mrimranqadir@hotmail.com

Muhammad Imran Qadir (Ed.)
All rights reserved-© 2020 Bentham Science Publishers

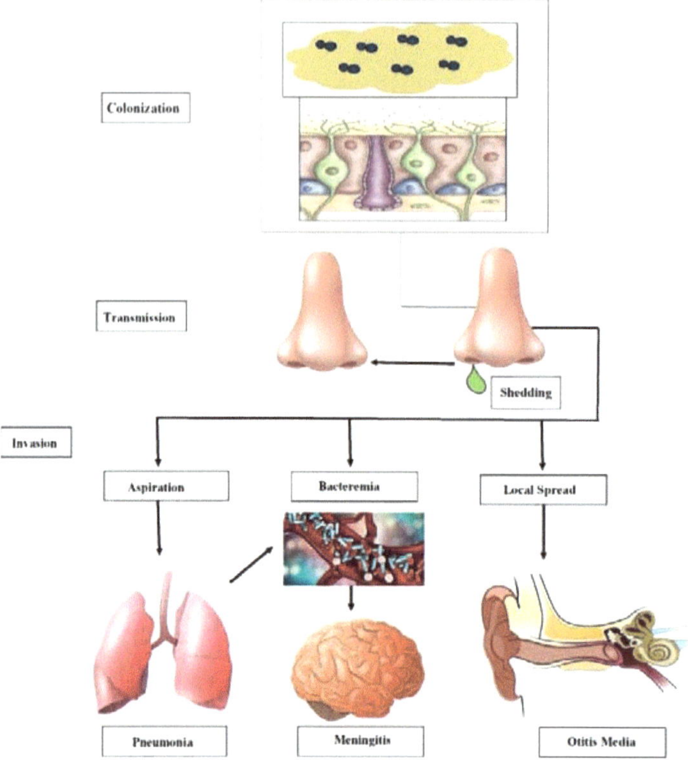

Fig. (2). Pneumonia pathogenesis.

SYMPTOMS

Common symptoms of pneumonia are:

- Cough with mucus
- Sore throat
- Chills
- Fever
- Pain in chest
- Fast breathing
- Shortness of breath

Symptoms of pneumonia can vary from mild to lethal. Further symptoms depend on the cause of the infection and its severity. Age and overall fitness of the individual also play a key role. As seen in Children, they don't have chest infection instead they suffer from high fever which becomes lethal and causes death. Similarly, older persons show different symptoms. In most cases, cold followed by the fever of 104°F high and cough with mucus observed as initial symptoms of pneumonia [4].

Certain symptoms are relevant to the site of infection. For example, if air passages become infected cough with sputum is a predominant symptom. In some cases, the spongy tissue that contains the air sacs in the lungs is infected. In this situation, the lungs become stiff due to impaired blood oxygenation causes the difficulty in breathing. Pneumonia that depends on the causative bacterium has a slow onset of symptoms. A deteriorating cough, severe headaches, and pain in muscles may be the symptoms [5].

DIAGNOSIS

Pneumonia can be diagnosed by:

- Chest X-ray
- Blood test
- Sputum test
- Urine test
- Pulse oximetry
- Fluid sample test
- Bronchoscopy

Initially, a doctor hears abnormal, crackling sounds in the chest and then recommends a chest X-ray that confirms the infection. Pneumonia can be detected by sputum culture test, sputum samples observed under the microscope for identification of microorganisms. In some situations, the detection of pneumonia caused by *Legionella Pneumococcus* determines by urine tests. Blood tests reveal the immune response of the body to certain infections. (WBCs) white blood cells count through a blood test that often gives a clue about the severity and cause of pneumonia. Pulse oximetry is a method in which an oxygen sensor is positioned on 1 of the patient's fingers. It shows whether lungs properly move enough oxygen into the bloodstream. A urine test can detect *Streptococcus pneumoniae* and *Legionella pneumophila* bacteria [6].

If a doctor suspects liquid in the pleural space of the chest, the fluid sample test is done by taking fluid through a needle inserted between ribs. This test helps to detect the cause of infection.

Bronchoscopy test considers the air passages of lungs. This is done by using a camera attached at one end of a flexible, thin tube which introduced into the mouth/nose. It enables the doctor to examine the throat and lungs. Doctors do this test when primary signs are severe and the body isn't properly responding to antibiotics [7].

MANAGEMENT

Antibiotics are used to treat pneumonia caused by bacteria. In severe cases, the affected person is usually referred to as the hospital. Oxygen therapy may be used if oxygen levels are low. Penicillin, Augmentin, Erythromycin, Amoxicillin are some common antibiotics used for *Streptococcus pneumoniae* infection. 2nd and 3rd generation antibiotics like cephalosporins, fluoroquinolones are used in *Klebsiella pneumoniae* infection. Macrolides *e.g.* erythromycin, azithromycin, and fluoroquinolones are some commonly used antibiotics for the treatment of Mycoplasma pneumonia. Fluoroquinolones are used to treat infection caused by *Legionella pneumoniae*.

A recent study in the Netherlands verified that the addition of steroid medication, dexamethasone, to antibiotic therapy reduces the period of hospitalization. This should be used for patients who have a compromised immune system.

Some antibiotics injected into a vein intravenously [8].

Vaccines are also available to treat pneumococcal infection. Two vaccines are (i) the pneumococcal conjugate vaccine (PCV13) (ii) the pneumococcal polysaccharide vaccine (PPV23; Pneumovax).

The pneumococcal conjugate vaccine is suggested for children and adults with age up to 64 years having chronic lung disease and diabetes-like health issues. The pneumococcal polysaccharide vaccine is suggested for those adults who have a greater risk of developing pneumococcal pneumonia-like people who have diabetes, alcoholic persons, smokers, and those persons whose spleen have been removed. According to the National Institutes of Health, vaccines against pneumonia do not prevent all symptoms. But it causes milder illness and reduces the risk of complications.

Respiratory therapy uses various techniques, including the delivery of the specific drug directly into the lungs. Oxygen therapy helps to maintain the bloodstream oxygen level. Oxygen is supplied through a nasal tube or a face mask. In extreme situations, a ventilator (a machine that supports breathing) may be used [9].

There are some preventive measures to reduce the risk of pneumonia, quit smoking because it makes the respiratory tract more susceptible to infection, like pneumonia. Washing hands properly with soap, disposing of used tissues, and cover coughs and sneezes may prevent pneumonia. Adaptation of a healthy lifestyle, proper sleep, a healthy diet, and exercise strengthens the immune system.

CONSENT FOR PUBLICATION

Not applicable.

CONFLICT OF INTEREST

The authors declare no conflict of interest, financial or otherwise.

ACKNOWLEDGEMENTS

Declared none.

REFERENCES

[1]   Schauner S, Erickson C, Fadare K, Stephens K. Community-acquired pneumonia in children: a look at the IDSA guidelines. J Fam Pract 2013; 62(1): 9-15.
[PMID: 23326817]

[2]   DeAntonio R, Yarzabal J-P, Cruz JP, Schmidt JE, Kleijnen J. Epidemiology of community-acquired pneumonia and implications for vaccination of children living in developing and newly industrialized countries: A systematic literature review. Hum Vaccin Immunother 2016; 12(9): 2422-40.
[http://dx.doi.org/10.1080/21645515.2016.1174356] [PMID: 27269963]

[3]   Gilani Z, Kwong YD, Levine OS, Deloria-Knoll M, Scott JAG, O'Brien KL, *et al.* A literature review and survey of childhood pneumonia etiology studies: 2000–2010. Clinical infectious diseases 2012; 54(suppl_2): S102-8.

[4]   Metlay JP, Schulz R, Li Y-H, *et al.* Influence of age on symptoms at presentation in patients with community-acquired pneumonia. Arch Intern Med 1997; 157(13): 1453-9.
[http://dx.doi.org/10.1001/archinte.1997.00440340089009] [PMID: 9224224]

[5]   Attridge RT, Frei CR. Health care-associated pneumonia: an evidence-based review. Am J Med 2011; 124(8): 689-97.
[http://dx.doi.org/10.1016/j.amjmed.2011.01.023] [PMID: 21663884]

[6]   Lynch T, Bialy L, Kellner JD, *et al.* A systematic review on the diagnosis of pediatric bacterial pneumonia: when gold is bronze. PLoS One 2010; 5(8)e11989
[http://dx.doi.org/10.1371/journal.pone.0011989] [PMID: 20700510]

[7]   Dockrell DH, Whyte MKB, Mitchell TJ. Pneumococcal pneumonia: mechanisms of infection and resolution. Chest 2012; 142(2): 482-91.
[http://dx.doi.org/10.1378/chest.12-0210] [PMID: 22871758]

[8]   Goyet S, Barennes H, Libourel T, van Griensven J, Frutos R, Tarantola A. Knowledge translation: a case study on pneumonia research and clinical guidelines in a low- income country. Implement Sci 2014; 9(1): 82.
[http://dx.doi.org/10.1186/1748-5908-9-82] [PMID: 24969242]

[9]   Pletz MW, Rohde GG, Welte T, Kolditz M, Ott S. Advances in the prevention, management, and treatment of community-acquired pneumonia. F1000 Res 2016; 5: 5.
[http://dx.doi.org/10.12688/f1000research.7657.1] [PMID: 26998243]

CHAPTER 3

Bacterial Tooth Decay: *Streptococcus mutans* is the Major Cause

Muhammad Imran Qadir[*] and **Shaiza Ali**

Institute of Molecular Biology & Biotechnology, Bahauddin Zakariya University, Multan, Pakistan

Abstract: Tooth decay is actually the destruction of the hard tissues of the tooth. This is caused by the acid attack due to the fermentation of carbohydrates due to bacterial attack by the bacterial species which colonize the mouth. *Streptococcus mutans* is the major cause of tooth decay. It occurs in different percentages in children of different ages. It is characterized by difficulty while eating, chewing, and even smiling. Clinical, radiographic, and technology-based methods are mainly used for the diagnosis of tooth decay.

Keywords: Bacterial Fermentation, Dental Decay, *Streptococcus mutans*.

INTRODUCTION

Tooth decay usually refers to the destruction of the dental hard tissues due to the acidic by-products which are produced due to the bacterial fermentation of the dietary carbohydrates. It is a chronic disease and it progresses slowly in most people. The surface of the tooth loses its tooth minerals due to the action of acids formed due to the bacteria after the ingestion of food which contains fermentable carbohydrates. When fermentable carbohydrates are taken in food and are eaten frequently they result in a decrease in pH and results in the loss of minerals from tooth [1].

CAUSES

The mouth is colonized by different types of bacterial species but few of them participate is dental decay. Dental decay is caused when solubilization of teeth occurs due to the accumulation of acid produced by certain types of bacteria in the mouth. Enterococci were the first bacteria that cause caries in gnotobiotic animals.

[*] **Corresponding author Muhammad Imran Qadir:** Institute of Molecular Biology and Biotechnology, Bahauddin Zakariya University, Multan, Pakistan; Tel: +92-61-9210071; Ext. 1920; Fax: +92-61-9210068; E-mail: mrimranqadir@hotmail.com

Muhammad Imran Qadir (Ed.)
All rights reserved-© 2020 Bentham Science Publishers

Actinomycetes are also found in the human mouth and they cause caries in hamsters [2]. *Streptococcus mutans* are the major cause of tooth decay. The genome of *mutans* UA159 has completely sequenced and is composed of 2,030,936 base pairs. The analysis of genome study showed that it has adaptations for the oral environment. *S. mutans* effect by metabolizing a wide range of carbohydrates [1].

PREVALENCE

Dental caries occurs about 23% in children aged from 2-6 years and about 56% are children aged 6-8 years. The prevalence of tooth decay is higher for Hispanic which is about 44% and for non-Hispanic blacks, the percentage is 44% which is compared with the non-Hispanic white children is about 31%. Non-Hispanic Asian children are likely to have dental caries [3].

SYMPTOMS

The tooth decay which occurs due to bacterial infection shows many symptoms which are followed by the experience of pain in the mouth, swelling in gums, pain while eating food or chewing, and even while smiling. Such that patients would not be able to eat easily. Bleeding from gums may also occur.

DIAGNOSIS

Clinical Methods

Visual detection of caries is the method most commonly used for the diagnosis of tooth decay. This method involves the oral examination which includes the cleaning and drying of the teeth and also the use of the explorers and also the use of visualizers to detect the area of concern. This process also helps in the detection of the area of the breakdown of the tooth.

Radiographic Methods

X-rays could also be used in dental applications. More recent developments include the higher-speed film and also the digital radiography. There are digital imaging techniques that could generate the image of the tooth and also the area of a breakdown of the tooth. The images of the teeth are obtained by the use of conventional films.

Technology-Based Methods

There are many other methods use for the diagnosis of tooth decay. Digital imaging is also used to detect the tooth surface. Polarized incident light is also used for diagnostic purposes. Fluorescence is also useful because of tooth fluoresce when exposed to ultraviolet rays [4].

MANAGEMENT

Fluoride is also effective in reducing the decay of the tooth. The major purpose of the use of fluoride is that dental caries is decreased. Fluoride is applied to the decaying part of the tooth.

The management of tooth decay involves the detection which follows checking the decay type and also the pathological changes. It also involves the monitoring of the lesion to determine whether the re-mineralization or the restoration treatment should be performed. Assessing each risk that is associated with tooth decay is also involved in the management. Last but not least monitoring of the follow-up patients periodically is also done [5].

CONSENT FOR PUBLICATION

Not applicable.

CONFLICT OF INTEREST

The authors declare no conflict of interest, financial or otherwise.

ACKNOWLEDGEMENTS

Declared none.

REFERENCES

[1]   Ajdić D, McShan WM, McLaughlin RE, *et al.* Genome sequence of Streptococcus mutans UA159, a cariogenic dental pathogen. Proc Natl Acad Sci USA 2002; 99(22): 14434-9.
        [http://dx.doi.org/10.1073/pnas.172501299] [PMID: 12397186]

[2]   Tanzer JM, Livingston J, Thompson AM. The microbiology of primary dental caries in humans. J Dent Educ 2001; 65(10): 1028-37.
        [http://dx.doi.org/10.1002/j.0022-0337.2001.65.10.tb03446.x] [PMID: 11699974]

[3]   Dye BA, Thornton-Evans G, Li X, Iafolla TJ. Dental caries and sealant prevalence in children and adolescents in the United States, 2011-2012. US Department of Health and Human Services, Centers for Disease Control and Prevention, National Center for Health Statistics 2015.

[4]   Zero DT, Fontana M, Martínez-Mier EA, *et al.* The biology, prevention, diagnosis and treatment of dental caries: scientific advances in the United States. J Am Dent Assoc 2009; 140 (Suppl. 1): 25S-34S.
        [http://dx.doi.org/10.14219/jada.archive.2009.0355] [PMID: 19723928]

[5]   Muntean A, Mesaros AS, Festila D, Mesaros M. Modern management of dental decay in children and adolescents - a review. Clujul Med 2015; 88(2): 137-9.
        [PMID: 26528061]

CHAPTER 4

Tuberculosis: A *Mycobacterium Tuberculosis* Infection

Muhammad Imran Qadir[*] and **Faryal Batool**

Institute of Molecular Biology & Biotechnology, Bahauddin Zakariya University, Multan, Pakistan

Abstract: Tuberculosis is a bacterial disease caused by *Mycobacterium tuberculosis* and can adversely affect the lungs and other parts of the body. It can be easily transmitted and can even cause death if not treated on time. In a report by WHO 10.4 million people were infected with TB in 2016. People with a weakened immune system, poverty, malnutrition are more susceptible to this disease. Different skin TST and blood tests IGRAs followed by chest radiography are conducted for diagnosis and confirmation of this disease. Antibiotics such as isoniazid, rifampicin, or rifapentine are prescribed in case of infection. BCG vaccine is effective for infants and not recommended for adults.

Keywords: Antibiotics, IGRAs, *Mycobacterium tuberculosis*, Weakened Immune System, Persistent Cough.

INTRODUCTION

Tuberculosis (TB) is among the deadliest disease caused by bacterium *Mycobacterium tuberculosis,* which can affect many body parts (Extrapulmonary TB) like lymph nodes, bones, spine, kidneys, and larynx, but most commonly lungs (Pulmonary TB). It can easily be transmitted to healthy people by coughing and sneezing near them. Inhalation of droplet nuclei from coughing and sneezing, in the air, enters from the mouth or nasal openings, passing through upper respiratory tract and bronchi, reaches the alveoli of the lungs. It affects approximately 10 million people every year but with timely diagnosis and proper treatment, it can be cured. One in three persons is known to be infected with this disease. According to a WHO Global Tuberculosis Report 2017, Tb is ranked 9th in death-causing diseases worldwide, and 10.4 million people infected in 2016 (10% are HIV co-infected) [1]. HIV patients are more susceptible to this disease

[*] **Corresponding author Muhammad Imran Qadir:** Institute of Molecular Biology and Biotechnology, Bahauddin Zakariya University, Multan, Pakistan; Tel: +92-61-9210071; Ext. 1920; Fax: +92-61-9210068; E-mail: mrimranqadir@hotmail.com

Muhammad Imran Qadir (Ed.)
All rights reserved © 2020 Bentham Science Publishers

as compared to other risk factors, for example, malnutrition, age (in the context of a weak immune system of very young and very old ones), *etc.* 1n 2016, 374000 deaths were reported among HIV positive TB patients. Over the last ten years, significant progress has been made to reduce the infection and mortality rate. 35% and 20% reduction in mortality and TB incidence was reported as compared to the data of 2015 [2].

SYMPTOMS

When infection starts and no symptoms appear, it is latent TB and it is called active TB when its symptoms appear Fig. (**3**) [3].

- A persistent cough that lasts for more than three weeks
- Weight loss
- Tiredness
- Fatigue
- Swelling of neck
- Fever
- Loss of appetite
- Chills
- Night sweats
- Chest pain

RISK FACTORS

Weak Immune System

People infected with different diseases, for example, HIV, cancers and chemotherapy, diabetes, kidney disease, *etc.* have weakened immune systems and such people are at high risk to be infected with TB [4].

Poverty and Malnutrition

Poor living conditions, lack of proper medical facilities, and malnutrition are some factors that can put people at high risk of TB.

Living in Areas which are at High Risk of Tuberculosis

People living in Asia, Russia, Africa, Caribbean Island, and Eastern Europe are at very high risk to be infected with TB.

PREVENTION OF TRANSMISSION

Some prevention guidelines for transmission of tuberculosis are mentioned below:

- Cover mouth and nose while coughing and sneezing.
- Washing of hands after coughing and sneezing.
- Isolation from office, schools, or workplaces.
- Less contact with unaffected people.

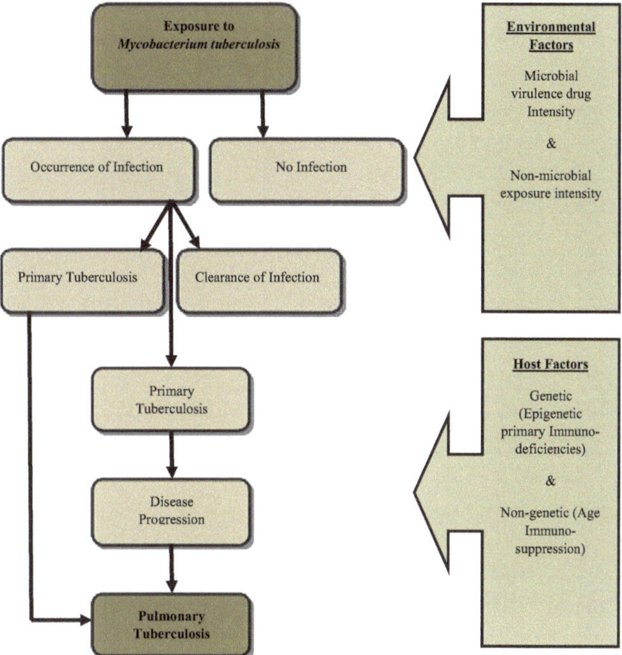

Fig. (3). Tuberculosis pathogenesis and factors affecting different phases of pathogenesis.

DIAGNOSIS

Different tests are used to diagnose TB and few of them are mentioned below:

Tuberculin Skin Test

TST is also known as Mantoux Test and most commonly used for latent TB [5]. In this test, a specific amount of PPD Tuberculin is injected into the skin of an arm. The red small and hard bump will appear on the spot of injection within 2 to 3 days if a person is infected with this disease due to sensitivity to PPD tuberculin [6]. If the prevalence of TB is high at that time, then the positive predictive value of the test will also be high. Incase to repeat the test, perform on another arm. This test is now considered outdated because of less specificity and sensitivity. In the case of Bacillus Calmette Guerin (BCG) vaccination skin will show mild response to the Mantoux test.

Sputum Smear Staining Test

A sample of sputum or phlegm is placed on the slide, stained with a dye, and washed with an acid solution, and slide is then examined under the microscope. If the cells retain the dye it means the test is positive. It is also known as Acid Fast Bacillus (AFB) because of the Mycobacteria which can strongly hold the dye even after washing with acid solution [7]. Sometimes bronchoscopy is also needed to obtain enough samples. This test was developed almost 100 years ago and according to WHO guidelines, for diagnosis of this disease, one positive result of the sputum smear test is required.

Interferon Gamma Release Assays Test (IGRAs)

IGRAs are one of the latest and accurate methods for TB diagnosis. In this test, INF-gamma released in response to antigens present in infection-causing bacteria are measured either by measuring IF-gamma concentration or by counting IFN-gamma secreting cells. There are two IFN-gamma release assays available, T-SPOT.TB and Quantiferon-TB Gold. This method is more specific as compared to TST but it can still not differentiate between active and latent TB [8].

Chest Radiography

A person infected with Tuberculosis will show some abnormal shadow on X-ray. Chest radiography locates the site of pathology and sometimes it is followed by sputum testing.

TREATMENT

Anti-tuberculosis drugs are usually preferred are isoniazid, pyrazinamide, ethambutol, and rifampicin. These are first-line drugs and preferred for newly diagnosed cases [9]. In the case of Drug resistance TB, four-second line drugs are prescribed, which include fluoroquinolone, ethionamide or prothionamide, parenteral agent, and cycloserine or para-aminosalicylic acid if cycloserine is not used [10]. For Latent TB isoniazid for six months but more preferably for nine months is prescribed. Isoniazid plus rifapentine weekly for three months or rifampin alone daily for four months or isoniazid plus rifampin daily for three months or isoniazid plus rifampin twice weekly for three months can be prescribed. 17 TB medicines are in clinical trials and soon to be commercialized in case of approval.

VACCINATION

Bacillus Calmette-Guerin (BCG) vaccine is commonly used to prevent TB in infants and it is not as effective in adults [6]. Before the vaccination, the Mantoux test is performed. About 12 vaccines are still in Phase I, Phase II, and Phase III trials.

CONSENT FOR PUBLICATION

Not applicable.

CONFLICT OF INTEREST

The authors declare no conflict of interest, financial or otherwise.

ACKNOWLEDGEMENTS

Declared none.

REFERENCES

[1]   Gilpin C, Korobitsyn A, Migliori GB, Raviglione MC, Weyer K. The World Health Organization standards for tuberculosis care and management. Eur Respiratory Soc 2018.
        [http://dx.doi.org/10.1183/13993003.00098-2018]

[2]   . Organization WH Global tuberculosis report 2016.

[3]   Wejse C, Gustafson P, Nielsen J, *et al.* TBscore: Signs and symptoms from tuberculosis patients in a low-resource setting have predictive value and may be used to assess clinical course. Scand J Infect Dis 2008; 40(2): 111-20.
        [http://dx.doi.org/10.1080/00365540701558698] [PMID: 17852907]

[4]   Melsew YA, Doan TN, Gambhir M, Cheng AC, McBryde E, Trauer JM. Risk factors for infectiousness of patients with tuberculosis: a systematic review and meta-analysis. Epidemiol Infect 2018; 146(3): 345-53.
        [http://dx.doi.org/10.1017/S0950268817003041] [PMID: 29338805]

[5]   Drobniewski FA, Caws M, Gibson A, Young D. Modern laboratory diagnosis of tuberculosis. Lancet Infect Dis 2003; 3(3): 141-7.
        [http://dx.doi.org/10.1016/S1473-3099(03)00544-9] [PMID: 12614730]

[6]   Tsai K-S, Chang H-L, Chien S-T, *et al.* Childhood tuberculosis: epidemiology, diagnosis, treatment, and vaccination. Pediatr Neonatol 2013; 54(5): 295-302.
        [http://dx.doi.org/10.1016/j.pedneo.2013.01.019] [PMID: 23597517]

[7]   Datta S, Shah L, Gilman RH, Evans CA. Comparison of sputum collection methods for tuberculosis diagnosis: a systematic review and pairwise and network meta-analysis. Lancet Glob Health 2017; 5(8): e760-71.
        [http://dx.doi.org/10.1016/S2214-109X(17)30201-2] [PMID: 28625793]

[8]   Liu Z, Zhang Q, Li Q, Wang L, Ren L. Application of interferon-γ release assay in extrapulmonary tuberculosis diagnosis, T-lymphocyte regulation, and efficacy evaluation in Northwest China. Int J Clin Exp Pathol 2017; 10: 3885-94.

[9]   Horsburgh CR Jr, Barry CE III, Lange C. Treatment of Tuberculosis. N Engl J Med 2015; 373(22): 2149-60.
        [http://dx.doi.org/10.1056/NEJMra1413919] [PMID: 26605929]

[10]   Organization WH, Initiative ST. Treatment of tuberculosis: guidelines. World Health Organization 2010.

CHAPTER 5

Leptospirosis: An Infection Which Leads to Kidney & Liver Damage

Muhammad Imran Qadir[*] and **Ghalia Batool Alvi**

Institute of Molecular Biology & Biotechnology, Bahauddin Zakariya University, Multan, Pakistan

Abstract: Leptospirosis is a bacterial disease caused by *Leptospira interrogans* which affects humans as well as animals. It can be transmitted from animals to humans in different ways. Global mortality and morbidity data indicate that of almost 1 million cases nearly 60,000 die each year. The agent responsible for this disease is common in tropical regions and the most suitable time for its growth is summer. People working with animals are more likely to contract this disease. It involves some flu-like symptoms: fever, diarrhea, cough, and severe pain. It can also damage the liver and kidneys and can also be fatal. Several methods have been devised for its diagnosis and mostly used methods are gene-based and serological. The main treatment of this disease is the use of antibiotics or a mix of antibiotics depending upon the status of the disease. Prevention from this disease is important as it can even cause death.

Key Words: Antibiotics, Kidney & Liver damage, Leptospirosis, *Leptospira interrogans*.

INTRODUCTION

Leptospirosis is a widely spread anthropozoonotic disease (a disease that can be transferred from animals to humans) mainly caused through a bacterium *Leptospira interrogans* [1]. Leptospires belong to phylum spirochetes. They are of two types: Saprophytes (non-pathogenic) and Pathogenic leptospires. These pathogenic leptospires are responsible for causing an infection known as Leptospirosis [2]. The natural host for leptospires are mammals, and they live in the proximal renal tubes of the host's kidney [3]. When these hosts urinate, then they are excreted out along with urine and can survive up to several months depending upon the environmental conditions. The urine of the infected mammals can contaminate soil, standing water, rivers, and streams. Humans always acquire

[*] **Corresponding author Muhammad Imran Qadir:** Institute of Molecular Biology and Biotechnology, Bahauddin Zakariya University, Multan, Pakistan; Tel: +92-61-9210071; Ext. 1920; Fax: +92-61-9210068; E-mail: mrimranqadir@hotmail.com

Muhammad Imran Qadir (Ed.)
All rights reserved-© 2020 Bentham Science Publishers

Leptospirosis from other animals like rats, pigs, dogs, and cattle, *etc.* by the direct interaction with these animals, from their excreted urine, from the environment in which they excrete their waste, *etc* [4]. This bacterium enters into the human body through open or wounded skin and mucosal membranes and if not treated may result in kidney and liver failure, meningitis, respiratory distress, and even fatal. Commonly, Leptospirosis is a disease of rural areas, but now even severe cases have reported in urban areas [5].

GLOBAL MORBIDITY AND MORTALITY

It was estimated in 2015 that yearly there were 1.03 million cases of Leptospirosis and about 58,900 patients died per annum because of this lethal infection. Mostly tropical regions had the highest morbidity and mortality rate around the world, *i.e.* countries located between the tropical regions of Cancer and Capricorn had about 73% of the incident and death rate. Men with 20-29 years age had the highest incident rate which was about 35.27/100,000, while men with 50-59 years age had the highest death rate, *i.e.* 2.89/100,000. Most of the morbidity and mortality cases of Leptospirosis were from the South and Southeast Asia, East Sub-Saharan Africa, Andean, Oceania, Central, and Tropical Latin America and the Caribbean [6].

Etiology

Several threats are linked with the occurrence of Leptospirosis. Depending upon the environmental conditions leptospires can be present anywhere.

Geographical Location

It is the most important factor as the highest morbidity and mortality rates were found in tropical regions. So, people living in those areas have the highest chances of developing Leptospirosis. Some other countries like South and Southeast Asia, East Sub-Saharan Africa, Andean, Oceania, Central, and Tropical Latin America and the Caribbean have the highest incidence and death rates [6].

Temperature

Temperature also decides the presence and absence of this infectious bacterium *Leptospira interrogans.* The most suitable temperature for the survival of this bacterium is summer in a rainy season. After rainfall, the standing water is the best habitat for this bacterium to survive [7].

Professional Activities

Professional activities can also become a risk factor if an individual is working in a place where he/she is in direct contact with the animals. As animals are the highest reservoirs of this bacterium so working with animals can end you having Leptospirosis. Dairy farmers, abattoir workers, veterinary employees, *etc.* are at the highest risk of developing Leptospirosis because they can acquire this disease after animal biting, contact with contaminated urine, contact with animal blood, and during the time of milking. Also, those individuals who have the chances of contact with rodents are at high risk like miners, rodent controllers, foresters, workers in a sewer system, hunters, fish farm workers, soldiers, *etc.*

Pet Animals

Having pets like dogs, cats can also act as a risk factor for developing Leptospirosis Fig. (**4**). Although the risk is not as higher in cats as with other mammals like dogs, but still they are capable of causing Leptospirosis. The level of risk also depends upon the sanitary conditions of the pets and their separation from possible sources of Leptospires.

Wounded Skin

Open or wounded skin can also make you vulnerable to Leptospires. The normal route of entry of this bacterium is through the wounded or cracked skin. So, wounded or punctured skin increases the chances of the entry of the pathogen into the body resulting in infection [8].

SYMPTOMS OF LEPTOSPIROSIS

There are several symptoms associated with Leptospirosis. Most of its symptoms match flu, which is the reason that sometimes it is misunderstood as flu. There are two stages of Leptospirosis:

The First Stage is known as an acute stage. It is also called as Septicemia. Its duration is about 3-10 days. Symptoms associated with this stage are:

- High Fever
- Myalgia (muscle aches)
- Diarrhea
- Cough
- Abdominal Pain
- Headache
- Nausea and Vomiting
- Chills
- Skin Rashes
- Redness of Eyes

• Jaundice [4]

The Second Stage which is also known as the Immune Stage is much more severe than the first stage and it may even prove fatal if not treated [4]. Major Symptoms associated with the immune stage are:

• Kidney Failure
• Liver Failure
• Meningitis (Swelling of the defensive membranes of Brain and Spinal Cord) [9].

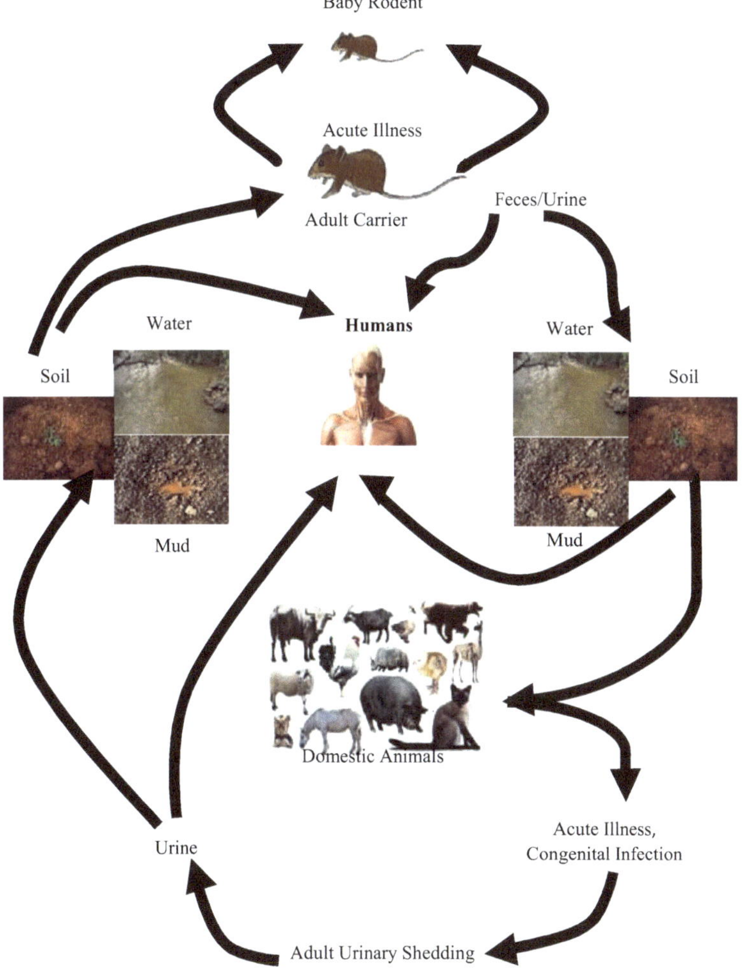

Fig. (4). Life Cycle of Leptospirosis.

DIAGNOSIS OF LEPTOSPIROSIS

Diagnosis of Leptospirosis is a very critical step and has to be done with care because the existence of disease and treatment is decided after diagnosis. Different techniques have been developed including direct microscopy, gene-based and serological methods.

Direct Microscopic Examination

Direct microscopic examination of Leptospirosis is done, if possible. The agent responsible for this disease is observable under dark-field microscopy due to its size of 6 to 20 μm in length and 0.15 μm diameter. Usually, 10^2 to 10^7 of the pathogen is detected in one ml of blood or urine in the acute stage [10]. The threshold of this technique is usually 10^4.

Gene-Based Techniques

Several genetic techniques are available for the detecting or diagnosis of leptospirosis.

Polymerase Chain Reaction

In this technique, the DNA of the causative agent of leptospirosis is amplified using PCR. Usually, Real-Time PCR is used because it gives swift results which are most likely error-free. The PCR can detect even the small amount of leptospires 10 to 100 in one ml of blood or even urine [11].

Isothermal Techniques

The isothermal technique is a kind of variant of PCR. A thermal cycler is used in PCR while a simple heating unit is sufficient to carry out the isothermal technique. This method involves the detection of a 16s rRNA of leptospires using its relevant primers. This technique has been applied for the detection of the pathogenic agent in urine [12].

Serological Methods

Different serological methods used in the diagnosis of leptospirosis are given below.

Microscopic Agglutination Test (MAT)

It is one of the oldest techniques devised for the diagnosis of leptospirosis. This technique involves the agglutination of antigens of leptospire bacteria with the antigens produced host's immune system. Different serial dilutions of serum of hosts are prepared and are incubated by adding antigens of different strains of leptospires. The dilution which shows 50% or more agglutination under dark-field microscopy refers to the existence of the disease in the host [4].

Elisa

This is another widely used method for the diagnosis of leptospirosis. IgM or IgG Elisa kit is used in this method. If the causative agent is present in the host's body, then antibodies are present in the host's blood. Elisa is performed using the host's serum and if antibodies are present, then it leads to a positive diagnosis of leptospirosis through Elisa [13].

Other Techniques

Several other methods have been devised for the diagnosis of leptospirosis. These include hem-agglutination, macro-agglutination, indirect-immunofluorescence, and many others. But these approaches are hardly used due to their limitations of specificity and efficiency [4].

TREATMENT

The selection of the treatment entirely relies upon the current condition and symptoms of the disease. Patient with acute stage having mild symptoms like flu, fever, headache, *etc.* do not require high profile vaccines instead they only need Symptomatic treatment (treatment based on the symptoms not on the cause of the disease), but if these mild symptoms lead to some severe symptoms like jaundice they need to be properly treated [14].

Antibiotic Therapy is the basic treatment for Leptospirosis as it is a bacterial disease. In some cases, after 2-4 days of infection, antibiotic therapy reduced the extent of infection. Also in a patient with severe conditions, the administration of antibiotics has shown clinically efficient results and a clear reduction in mortality rates. Different types of antibiotics are efficient in Leptospirosis *e.g.* Ampicillin, Ofloxoacin, Amoxicillin, Tetracycline, Clarithromycin, Azithromycin, Penicillin, and Doxycycline, *etc.* Depending upon the severity of the disease, these antibiotics alone or mixed with one or two are given to the patients. In the case of mild infection, ampicillin and amoxicillin are given to the patient. Penicillin G and ampicillin are considered best in case of severe disease. Doxycycline is effective in both mild disease and prophylaxis. According to one study, ceftriaxone in combination with penicillin is also a possible treatment for acute severe Leptospirosis [9, 15].

In some countries, vaccines are also available to treat Leptospirosis and in other countries vaccine development is in large clinical trials. According to study in Cuba in clinical trials, not even a single side effect of the vaccine is observed but one problem is that these vaccines are developing from the killed strains of Leptospires and using a whole organism as a vaccine may cause adverse reactions and also it is not a sustainable treatment because these are short-term vaccines so, repeated vaccination is required which is not an advantage. Another disadvantage is that there is a possibility of developing the autoimmune disease as a side effect of these polyvalent vaccines [15, 16].

PREVENTIVE MEASURES

- Usage of open water or water from a swamp, canals, and lakes must be avoided because the agent responsible for Leptospirosis can be found in such contaminated water.
- Any of the wound or punctured skin must be treated as early as possible because it can act as an easy entrance for several pathogens.
- People dealing with animals must wear protective clothing to avoid contact with the agent.
- Rodents are also the source of this agent. Therefore, proper rodent control mechanisms should be adopted in houses.
- Animal waste must be dumped properly so that its contact with the human environment is least.
- People who pet animals must have a proper check-up of their pets regularly from the veterinarian.
- The use of a healthy diet is also advisable for humans because it helps in improving the immune system.

Caution

The major carriers of this pathogen are pets. Hence, regular check-up of animals by an authorized veterinarian is extremely important.

It is a fatal disease which may not be taken lightly. It can cause kidney damage, liver failure, respiratory tract problems, meningitis, and even death.

CONSENT FOR PUBLICATION

Not applicable.

CONFLICT OF INTEREST

The authors declare no conflict of interest, financial or otherwise.

ACKNOWLEDGEMENTS

Declared none.

REFERENCES

[1]   Johnson RC, Faine S. Leptospira. Keieg NR, Nolt JG Bergey's manual of systematic bacteriology 2nd Baltimore USA.. Williams &Wilkins 1984; pp. 62-7.

[2]   Michel V, Branger C, Andre-Fontaine G. Epidemiology of leptospirosis. Rev Cubana Med Trop 2002; 54(1): 7-10.
[PMID: 15846932]

[3]   Adler B, de la Peña Moctezuma A. Leptospira and leptospirosis. Vet Microbiol 2010; 140(3-4): 287-96.
[http://dx.doi.org/10.1016/j.vetmic.2009.03.012] [PMID: 19345023]

[4]   Picardeau M. Diagnosis and epidemiology of leptospirosis. Med Mal Infect 2013; 43(1): 1-9.
[http://dx.doi.org/10.1016/j.medmal.2012.11.005] [PMID: 23337900]

[5]   Yimer E, Koopman S, Messele T, Wolday D, Newayeselassie B, Gessesse N, *et al.* Human leptospirosis, in Ethiopia: a pilot study in Wonji. Ethiop J Health Dev 2017; 18(1) [EJHD].
[http://dx.doi.org/10.4314/ejhd.v18i1.9866]

[6]   Costa F, Hagan JE, Calcagno J, *et al.* Global morbidity and mortality of leptospirosis: a systematic review. PLoS Negl Trop Dis 2015; 9(9): e0003898.
[http://dx.doi.org/10.1371/journal.pntd.0003898] [PMID: 26379143]

[7]   Sakundarno M, Bertolatti D, Maycock B, Spickett J, Dhaliwal S. Risk factors for leptospirosis infection in humans and implications for public health intervention in Indonesia and the Asia-Pacific region. Asia Pac J Public Health 2014; 26(1): 15-32.
[http://dx.doi.org/10.1177/1010539513498768] [PMID: 24097928]

[8]   Wasiński B, Dutkiewicz J. Leptospirosis--current risk factors connected with human activity and the environment. Ann Agric Environ Med 2013; 20(2): 239-44.
[PMID: 23772568]

[9]   Plank R, Dean D. Overview of the epidemiology, microbiology, and pathogenesis of *Leptospira* spp. in humans. Microbes Infect 2000; 2(10): 1265-76.
[http://dx.doi.org/10.1016/S1286-4579(00)01280-6] [PMID: 11008116]

[10]   Musso D, La Scola B. Laboratory diagnosis of leptospirosis: a challenge. J Microbiol Immunol Infect 2013; 46(4): 245-52.
[http://dx.doi.org/10.1016/j.jmii.2013.03.001] [PMID: 23639380]

[11]   Levett PN, Morey RE, Galloway RL, Turner DE, Steigerwalt AG, Mayer LW. Detection of pathogenic leptospires by real-time quantitative PCR. J Med Microbiol 2005; 54(Pt 1): 45-9.
[http://dx.doi.org/10.1099/jmm.0.45860-0] [PMID: 15591254]

[12]   Koizumi N, Nakajima C, Harunari T, *et al.* A new loop-mediated isothermal amplification method for rapid, simple, and sensitive detection of Leptospira spp. in urine. J Clin Microbiol 2012; 50(6): 2072-4.
[http://dx.doi.org/10.1128/JCM.00481-12] [PMID: 22422858]

[13]   Terpstra WJ, Ligthart GS, Schoone GJ. ELISA for the detection of specific IgM and IgG in human leptospirosis. J Gen Microbiol 1985; 131(2): 377-85.
[PMID: 3981131]

[14]   Levett PN. Leptospirosis. Clin Microbiol Rev 2001; 14(2): 296-326.
[http://dx.doi.org/10.1128/CMR.14.2.296-326.2001] [PMID: 11292640]

[15]   Bharti AR, Nally JE, Ricaldi JN, *et al.* Leptospirosis: a zoonotic disease of global importance. Lancet

Infect Dis 2003; 3(12): 757-71.
[http://dx.doi.org/10.1016/S1473-3099(03)00830-2] [PMID: 14652202]

[16]   Ko AI, Goarant C, Picardeau M. Leptospira: the dawn of the molecular genetics era for an emerging
       zoonotic pathogen. Nat Rev Microbiol 2009; 7(10): 736-47.
       [http://dx.doi.org/10.1038/nrmicro2208] [PMID: 19756012]

CHAPTER 6

Syphilis: A Disease Which Spreads Through Sexual Contact

Muhammad Imran Qadir[*] and **Rabia Hussain**

Institute of Molecular Biology & Biotechnology, Bahauddin Zakariya University, Multan, Pakistan

Abstract: Syphilis is an infectious disease caused by a bacterial strain named as *Treponema pallidum* and is spread through sexual contacts with the infected person, blood transfusion, and sharing of syringes with the infected person. The symptoms of this disease include an outgrowth on the skin, dizziness, skin rashes, irritation, and even stroke in severe cases. This disease is diagnosed both by using non-Treponema tests and by specific-Treponema tests. Culturing of the sample taken from the rash or outgrowth is also very helpful to diagnose the presence of infectious entities. It is a curable disease and is easily cured by a short term course of antibiotics. Another method to cure this disease is the use of penicillin injection after the regular interval of time. This chapter summarized the causing agent, symptoms, commonly used diagnostic tests and management strategies to cure this disease.

Keywords: Cure, Rapid Syphilis Test, Rapid Plasma Reagin Test, Syphilis, *Treponema pallidum*, Symptoms.

INTRODUCTION

Syphilis is an infectious disease that is transmitted by sexual contacts to an infected person. This disease is caused by the bacteria named *Treponema pallidum*. Syphilis is spread by sexual contacts with the infected person, by blood transfusion, by sharing injections and also transmitted from an infected mother to the child during pregnancy. By sharing clothes, bathrooms, cutlery with the diseased person there is no chance to be infected. In 2006 roundabout 9.7 million small children less than 5 years old and almost 4 million neonatal Childs were died off due to this disease in developing countries. There is 3.2 million infected childbirth globally, which includes more than 90% of children belong to developing countries. In Africa there is an estimate that 2.7% of pregnant women are infected with this disease indicates that round about 900,000 pregnancies at ri-

[*] **Corresponding author Muhammad Imran Qadir:** Institute of Molecular Biology and Biotechnology, Bahauddin Zakariya University, Multan, Pakistan; Tel: +92-61-9210071; Ext. 1920; Fax: +92-61-9210068; E-mail: mrimranqadir@hotmail.com

Muhammad Imran Qadir (Ed.)
All rights reserved-© 2020 Bentham Science Publishers

sk each year. Syphilis in the pregnancy become a serious global health burden with adverse outcomes, for example, infant mortality. Approximately 3.6 million Childs are affected due to infected or diseased mothers each year.

The medical cost for this disease is about 309 million dollars [1]. According to the world health organization, approximately 700,000-1.5 million people with this disease were reported in 2004. Roundabout 45-70% of the infected person catches this disease from the infected mother. This disease causes 420,000-600,000 death out of which 40% includes stillbirth and 20% includes neonatal deaths [2]. WHO estimates that 2 million women are infected due to syphilis annually, most of the carrier pregnant women belonged to low/middle income countries. Roundabout 69% of untreated pregnant women show severe pregnancy outcomes such as stillbirth results in about 25% cases, neonatal death results in about 11% cases, infected childbirth results in 20% cases, and low birth-weight childbirth results in 13% cases [3]. According to the CDC report related to STD, there were only 5979 syphilis cases reported in the U.S out of which 59% were male and 41% female victims. The gradual increase in cases day by day, including 8724 cases in 2005, 13774 cases in 2010, and 19999 in 2014 out of which 91% were male and only 9% were female in the USA.

SYMPTOMS

Syphilis is divided into three categories based on their symptoms named primary syphilis, secondary syphilis, and tertiary syphilis. The first symptoms of syphilis appeared after 10 days-3 weeks of infection. The most common symptoms of primary syphilis include the painless sore that appears on the point at which an infectious entity is transmitted usually on the vagina and penis. That sore disappeared in about 2-6 weeks after infection. If the infection remains untreated then it causes the secondary stage of syphilis. Symptoms of secondary syphilis start after few weeks of the disappearance of sore and these include a non-itchy rash of the skin, tiredness, joint pains, headaches, fever, small skin outgrowths on the vulva in the woman's case and around the anus in the case of both men and women, hair loss, swollen lymph glands, and weight loss. These symptoms also disappear after a few weeks, or in months. Without any treatment, syphilis becomes 'latent' and no symptoms appear at all, but the infection is there. This stage could be happened for years in some cases even for decades and known as tertiary syphilis. Common symptoms of syphilis include dementia, paralysis, heart diseases, loss of coordination, deafness, stroke, blindness, numbness and skin rashes, *etc.* Tertiary syphilis also causes death in some cases so it is important to go to the healthcare center and properly examined by the professionals.

DIAGNOSIS

To diagnose syphilis first basic way is the physical examination by a doctor or nurse who will ask to examine genitals in case of male and inside the vagina in the case of women and a physical examination of other parts of the body to check for growths or rashes on the skin may be caused due to syphilis. Another way is to test blood which shows that either infectious agent of this disease is present in the body or not, either this disease present in the past or not. Blood test for a few weeks is done at regular intervals then accurate results could be obtained. Another way to check out the presence of syphilis is the swab test for which a swab is used to take a sample of fluid from any sores and after culturing of this sample it can be checked either syphilis causing agents are present or not. Syphilis is an important health issue in mostly low-income countries because these have limited or no capacity for testing and mostly rely on the non- specific Treponema test. According to the recent development of a new rapid Treponema, tests can increase the screening process where traditional tests are not available due to any reason. According to recent studies ICS syphilis tests which is a newly developed test have high sensitivity of about 0·86 median and 0.75-0.94 interquartile range. This test also has a higher specificity as compared to the non-specific Treponema test. And further research evaluating the ICS tests, in primary syphilis cases and among the patients infected with HIV is also effective in syphilis screening programs. ICS syphilis tests are easy to perform, economic in range, and there is no need to be refrigerated and no need to highly trained laboratory professionals for carrying out the test [4]. Another study highlights the importance of a point-of-care syphilis test which has high accuracy, simple to use and has the potential to increase the coverage of antenatal screening. This study also suggests that the use of ICS tests for antenatal screening of syphilis disease is highly cost-effective in low-income countries such as Africa with a reduction in disability-adjusted life years [5]. An assessment by Bonawitz suggests that recently developed rapid syphilis tests commonly abbreviated as RST have a high sensitivity of about 85.7%-100% and specificity of about 96%-100% and these tests do not require the traditional laboratory infrastructure that is usually required to carry out rapid plasma regain test commonly abbreviated as RPR test [6]. Another study by Owusu-Edusei of 1000 pregnant women in the population having a high prevalence of syphilis disease was done. He develops a model which is based on the comparison between health and economic outcomes of traditional tests for the detection of syphilis such as rapid plasma regain anti- *Treponema pallidum* assay abbreviated as RPRTPHA and new tests such as dual point of care commonly known as dual-POC and ICS. He found out that ICS testing was the most cost-effective strategy after the dual-POC strategy [7]. Kuznik's study suggests that immune-chromatographic point-of-care tests are time-saving, reliable, simple to perform, inexpensive, and economically suitable for antenatal care settings [8]. A study carried out by Terris-Prestholt highlights that newly developed tests are time-saving as compared to the traditional RPR test. In traditional tests strategy was usually done in the form of batches and time was given to the patients of the next day or so. They concluded that most of the women never came for picking up the test results, even if they were positive. So this issue lacking the usefulness of RPR in ANC. He further highlighted the importance of rapid syphilis immune-chromatographic strips abbreviated as ICS and dual rapid syphilis tests commonly known as dual-RST [9].

MANAGEMENT

Syphilis is treated by the short course of antibiotics. The treatment type which is needed depends on the period of the syphilis disease. Syphilis that last for two years is commonly treated with the injection of penicillin into buttocks. The antibiotic course for 10-14 days is used to cure this disease if penicillin is not available. Syphilis lasted for two years or more than 2 years is commonly treated with the 3 penicillin injections into buttocks given after the period of a weak. An alternative antibiotic tablet treatment course for 28 days is recommended if penicillin is not available. To avoid the dangerous effect of this disease, any sexual activity and close sexual contact with a person are avoided until two weeks after the treatment finishes. Another analysis which is done by Kuznik concluded that the adverse result of pregnancy-associated with syphilis can be prevented when an infected mother is identified and treated before the third trimester [8]. Bowen *et al.* found that in pregnant women with syphilis who deliver after 20 weeks of gestation, treatment with penicillin is 98% effective at preventing congenital syphilis [10]. Penicillin is readily available, cheap, and highly effective against *Treponema pallidum* [11].

CONSENT FOR PUBLICATION

Not applicable.

CONFLICT OF INTEREST

The authors declare no conflict of interest, financial or otherwise.

ACKNOWLEDGEMENTS

Declared none.

REFERENCES

[1]   Kahn JG, Jiwani A, Gomez GB, *et al.* The cost and cost-effectiveness of scaling up screening and treatment of syphilis in pregnancy: a model. PLoS One 2014; 9(1): e87510.
[http://dx.doi.org/10.1371/journal.pone.0087510] [PMID: 24489931]

[2]   Krüger C, Malleyeck I. Congenital syphilis: still a serious, under-diagnosed threat for children in resource-poor countries. World J Pediatr 2010; 6(2): 125-31.
[http://dx.doi.org/10.1007/s12519-010-0028-z] [PMID: 20490768]

[3]   Hawkes S, Matin N, Broutet N, Low N. Effectiveness of interventions to improve screening for syphilis in pregnancy: a systematic review and meta-analysis. Lancet Infect Dis 2011; 11(9): 684-91.
[http://dx.doi.org/10.1016/S1473-3099(11)70104-9] [PMID: 21683653]

[4]   Tucker JD, Bu J, Brown LB, Yin Y-P, Chen X-S, Cohen MS. Accelerating worldwide syphilis screening through rapid testing: a systematic review. Lancet Infect Dis 2010; 10(6): 381-6.
[http://dx.doi.org/10.1016/S1473-3099(10)70092-X] [PMID: 20510278]

[5]   Kuznik A, Lamorde M, Nyabigambo A, Manabe YC. Antenatal syphilis screening using point-of-care testing in Sub-Saharan African countries: a cost-effectiveness analysis. PLoS Med 2013; 10(11)e1001545
[http://dx.doi.org/10.1371/journal.pmed.1001545] [PMID: 24223524]

[6]   Bonawitz RE, Duncan J, Hammond E, *et al.* Assessment of the impact of rapid syphilis tests on syphilis screening and treatment of pregnant women in Zambia. Int J Gynaecol Obstet 2015; 130(S1) (Suppl. 1): S58-62.
[http://dx.doi.org/10.1016/j.ijgo.2015.04.015] [PMID: 25968492]

[7]   Owusu-Edusei K Jr, Gift TL, Ballard RC. Cost-effectiveness of a dual non-treponemal/treponemal syphilis point-of-care test to prevent adverse pregnancy outcomes in sub-Saharan Africa. Sex Transm Dis 2011; 38(11): 997-1003.
[http://dx.doi.org/10.1097/OLQ.0b013e3182260987] [PMID: 21992974]

[8]   Kuznik A, Habib AG, Manabe YC, Lamorde M. Estimating the public health burden associated with adverse pregnancy outcomes resulting from syphilis infection across 43 countries in sub-Saharan Africa. Sex Transm Dis 2015; 42(7): 369-75.
[http://dx.doi.org/10.1097/OLQ.0000000000000291] [PMID: 26222749]

[9]   Terris-Prestholt F, Vickerman P, Torres-Rueda S, *et al.* The cost-effectiveness of 10 antenatal syphilis screening and treatment approaches in Peru, Tanzania, and Zambia. Int J Gynaecol Obstet 2015; 130(S1) (Suppl. 1): S73-80.
[http://dx.doi.org/10.1016/j.ijgo.2015.04.007] [PMID: 25963907]

[10]   Bowen V, Su J, Torrone E, Kidd S, Weinstock H. Increase in incidence of congenital syphilis - United States, 2012-2014. MMWR Morb Mortal Wkly Rep 2015; 64(44): 1241-5.
[http://dx.doi.org/10.15585/mmwr.mm6444a3] [PMID: 26562206]

[11]   Saloojee H, Velaphi S, Goga Y, Afadapa N, Steen R, Lincetto O. The prevention and management of congenital syphilis: an overview and recommendations. Bull World Health Organ 2004; 82(6): 424-30.
[PMID: 15356934]

CHAPTER 7

Leprosy: An Infection Which Leads Characterized by Granulomata

Muhammad Imran Qadir[*] and **Maleeha Batool**

Institute of Molecular Biology & Biotechnology, Bahauddin Zakariya University, Multan, Pakistan

Abstract: Leprosy is actually a disease that is said to be chronic and it is caused by a mycobacterium *Bacillus leprae*. It is related to physical or mental disablement and mainly it affects eyes, skin, peripheral nerves, and various organs. It is endemic to various domains of the world. Lesions appear on the body and the peripheral nerves become thick and tough which are the main symptoms of the disease. Thus, it can be diagnosed by performing a smear test or by a biopsy experiment. First-line drugs, second-line drugs, and various vaccines are available for the treatment of leprosy.

Keywords: *Bacillus leprae*, First-Line Drug, Leprosy, Peripheral Nerves, Smear Test.

INTRODUCTION

Leprosy or Hansen disease is a constant disease that is characterized by granulomata and the causal agent behind this disease is mycobacterium *Bacillus leprae*. A Norwegian physician named Gerhard Henrik Armauer Hansen identified this mycobacterium in the 19th century [1]. Leprosy is related to physical or mental unfitness. It mainly affects the skin and the nerves lying outside the brain and the spinal cord (peripheral nerves) and to this time indigenous in different domains of the world. Clinical demonstration of the disease relies upon the condition of the immune system of the patient during transmission and throughout the disease [2].

Leprosy programs that were enforced from 2006 to 2010 at the national levels had a positive outcome as they met up with the WHO's aim for the areas where leprosy is indigenous [3]. The written report of the prevalence of leprosy of about

[*] **Corresponding author Muhammad Imran Qadir:** Institute of Molecular Biology and Biotechnology, Bahauddin Zakariya University, Multan, Pakistan; Tel: +92-61-9210071; Ext. 1920; Fax: +92-61-9210068; E-mail: mrimranqadir@hotmail.com

Muhammad Imran Qadir (Ed.)
All rights reserved-© 2020 Bentham Science Publishers

212802 cases was given `in 2008. "Final push strategy" was given by the WHO in the early 1990s for leprosy having the open objective of elimination.

Countries like Mozambique and the Democratic Republic of the Congo reached the goal given by WHO, but many parts of the world remained highly prevalent by the disease [4].

SIGNS AND SYMPTOMS

The Peripheral nervous system is at first targeted by the *Bacillus leprae* which further leads to the huge range of clinical reflections that describe this infection from the mycobacterium. Peripheral nerves relating to the skin may be affected by lesions, mainly the medial, posterior tibial, lateral peroneal, and cubital nerves [5]. A perineural osteofibrosis response is a buildup that is not much deep, making the nerves capable of being perceived by the senses or mind at the time of physical examination. This nerve involvement gives rise to pain, thickening, and motor and sensory disablement [6]. Thickening of the outer or peripheral nerves is also there in many other diseases like primary amyloidosis and some other inheritable diseases (*e.g.*, Refsum diseases and Charcot-Marie-Tooth disease). Therefore there must be some kind of differential diagnosis. In most of the 95% of cases, it affects the musculoskeletal system [7] and [8]. Osteoporosis is the most significant and the second most usual sign observed in leprosy patients [9].

DIAGNOSIS

In 1997, WHO's proficient Committee on Leprosy set out the 3 fundamental signs based on which the disease is diagnosed clinically [2] and [10]. When a person who has not accomplished a course of medical care has one or more of these under mentioned signs, then the diagnosis is made.

These signs are:

1. The presence of a hypopigmented lesion on the skin
2. A tough or calloused peripheral nerve
3. A positive skin spot or presence of bacilli which have been discovered in a biopsy.

In case, all of these three signs are present in a person, then the symptomatic sensitivity has been said to be as serious as 97% [10]. The Smear test is performed mostly to diagnose the patients having the disease. This test is 100% specific and has 50% of the sensitivity. A smear is usually taken from an ear lobe, nasal mucosa, and/or from skin wounds [11, 12]. The stain that is used to make the mycobacterium visible is normally Ziehl-Neelsen stain. To interpret the results of the smear test, bacterial index or Ridley's logarithmic scale are used, which are registered as a number that comes after a plus sign to show the level of scarcity or richness of bacteria for each field.

MANAGEMENT

Leprosy is a risk to health worldwide. Its removal is feasible, as this contagious disease is one of those few diseases that meet definite but not specified or confined requirements for eradication. It can be spread by affected but untreated persons and thus can be diagnosed by using simple tools. Furthermore, impressive therapy is also present and once predominance falls below a specific point in a population, the probability of revival is not proximate. Eventually, contrary to tuberculosis, the infection got by leprosy does n't seem to be affected by HIV (human immunodeficiency virus) infection negatively. Thalidomide is the drug of choice, but sometimes clofazimine or prednisone can be recommended. In the early stages, the dosage for Thalidomide is 100 to 200mg/d, the remedy has perfectly retreated after three to four weeks [13, 14]. WHO presented multidrug therapy with clofazimine, dapsone, and rifampicin with the aim of first-line treatment in 1981. All of the patients must receive this drug under some proper supervision monthly. Clarithromycin, ofloxacin, and minocycline are among those drugs which have been used with the aim of second-line treatments. However, the duration of this treatment is long and shows logistical difficulties.

First-line Drugs

In first-line drugs, Rifampicin, which has been taken from Streptomyces fungi, has antibacterial action which is based on its ability to inhibit the synthesis of RNA. Quality of being poisonous to liver cells, vomiting, nausea, inflammation on the skin, and fever is this drug's major adverse effects. Clofazimine has low antibacterial activity. Although it is recognized to bind DNA, the mechanism of action of this drug is still not well understood. Clofazimine is related to the changes in colouring of the skin [15]. On the other hand, second-line drugs have been reported as highly active ones, but they bear high costs which prohibit employing them as the highest preference treatments.

Vaccines

Different vaccines have been proven efficient to one extent or another in some of the countries where leprosy has been reported as indigenous. The preventive consequence of a vaccine for leprosy is gained by adjusting the immune system in opposition to common mycobacterial antigens. The Convit vaccine was brought into existence in 1992, which is BCG (Bacillus Calmette-Guérin) in combination with Mycobacterium ICRC and M leprae. Other vaccines are based upon

Mycobacterium tufu which were suggested by Kalianina and Iushin in 1995 and one exploiting Mycobacterium habana. In some of the regions of the world, BCG vaccine is given to children whose age is under 12 years and who have some link with their relatives having leprosy.

CONSENT FOR PUBLICATION

Not applicable.

CONFLICT OF INTEREST

The authors declare no conflict of interest, financial or otherwise.

ACKNOWLEDGEMENTS

Declared none.

REFERENCES

[1]   Fitness J, Tosh K, Hill AV. Genetics of susceptibility to leprosy. Genes Immun 2002; 3(8): 441-53.
        [http://dx.doi.org/10.1038/sj.gene.6363926] [PMID: 12486602]

[2]   Lockwood DN, Saunderson PR. Nerve damage in leprosy: a continuing challenge to scientists, clinicians and service providers. Int Health 2012; 4(2): 77-85.
        [http://dx.doi.org/10.1016/j.inhe.2011.09.006] [PMID: 24029146]

[3]   José A, Soares CLR, Marchiori M. Lanza FdC, Corso SD, Malaguti C. The glittre-ADL test can be used to assess the functional performance in patients with leprosy: A controlled transversal study. Edorium Journal of Disability and Rehabilitation 2016; 2: 131-7.
        [http://dx.doi.org/10.5348/D05-2016-20-OA-16]

[4]   Gulia A, Fried I, Massone C. New insights in the pathogenesis and genetics of leprosy. F1000 Med Rep 2010; 2: 2.
        [http://dx.doi.org/10.3410/M2-30] [PMID: 20948855]

[5]   Sehgal VN, Sardana K, Dogra S. Management of complications following leprosy: an evolving scenario. J Dermatolog Treat 2007; 18(6): 366-74.
        [http://dx.doi.org/10.1080/09546630701364750] [PMID: 18058495]

[6]   Maki DD, Yousem DM, Corcoran C, Galetta SL. MR imaging of Dejerine-Sottas disease. AJNR Am J Neuroradiol 1999; 20(3): 378-80.
        [PMID: 10219400]

[7]   Faget G, Mayoral A. Bone changes in leprosy: A clinical and roentgenology study of 505 cases. Radiology 1944; 42(1): 1-13.
        [http://dx.doi.org/10.1148/42.1.1]

[8]   Chhabriya BD, Sharma NC, Bansal NK, Agrawal GR. Bone changes in leprosy. A study of 50 cases. Indian J Lepr 1985; 57(3): 632-9.
        [PMID: 3831105]

[9]   Tinoco F, Bismark J. Prevalencia de lepra y contagio de familiares o personas que estan en contacto con pacientes que tienen la enfermedad de hansen en el Cantón Atahualpa de la Provincia de el Oro periodo febrero-agosto 2011 2012.

[10]   Moschella SL. An update on the diagnosis and treatment of leprosy. J Am Acad Dermatol 2004; 51(3): 417-26.
[http://dx.doi.org/10.1016/j.jaad.2003.11.072] [PMID: 15337986]

[11]   Hatta M, van Beers SM, Madjid B, Djumadi A, de Wit MY, Klatser PR. Distribution and persistence of Mycobacterium leprae nasal carriage among a population in which leprosy is endemic in Indonesia. Trans R Soc Trop Med Hyg 1995; 89(4): 381-5.
[http://dx.doi.org/10.1016/0035-9203(95)90018-7] [PMID: 7570870]

[12]   Ramaprasad P, Fernando A, Madhale S, *et al.* Transmission and protection in leprosy: indications of the role of mucosal immunity. Lepr Rev 1997; 68(4): 301-15.
[http://dx.doi.org/10.5935/0305-7518.19970038] [PMID: 9503866]

[13]   Jakeman P, Smith WC. Thalidomide in leprosy reaction. Lancet 1994; 343(8895): 432-3.
[http://dx.doi.org/10.1016/S0140-6736(94)92686-7] [PMID: 7905950]

[14]   Heriberto V, Roberto A. Talidomida en dermatología. Revisión de sus orígenes, su actual redescubrimiento y sus nuevas aplicaciones. Dermatol Rev Mex 1998; 42: 252-65.

[15]   Vieira JLF, Riveira JGB, Martins AdeN, Silva JP, Salgado CG. Methemoglobinemia and dapsone levels in patients with leprosy. Braz J Infect Dis 2010; 14(3): 319-21.
[http://dx.doi.org/10.1590/S1413-86702010000300022] [PMID: 20835521]

CHAPTER 8

Burn Infection: *Pseudomonas Aeruginosa* and *Staphylococcus Aureus* are the Major Pathogens

Muhammad Imran Qadir[*] and **Momal Tariq**

Institute of Molecular Biology & Biotechnology, Bahauddin Zakariya University, Multan, Pakistan

Abstract: A burn is an injury to skin or tissues of the body caused by heat, electricity, cold, chemicals, and radiation. *Pseudomonas aeruginosa* (gram-negative bacteria) and methicillin-resistant *Staphylococcus aureus* (gram-positive bacteria) cause burn infections in humans. Burn causes breathing problems and redness of the skin, damage to blood vessels causes' skin to become black or brown with no blisters. Burn can be diagnosed by examination, depth of a wound, or its associated infections. In developed countries "treatment" cannot be difficult as much as in underdeveloped countries. This is because of lack of awareness or poor income in underdeveloped countries they depend on traditional treatment which left scars of a wound.

Key Words: Burn, Blisters, Injury.

INTRODUCTION

A burn is an injury to skin or tissues of the body caused by heat, electricity, cold, chemicals, and radiation. *Pseudomonas aeruginosa* (gram-negative bacteria) and methicillin-resistant *Staphylococcus aureus* (gram-positive bacteria) cause burn infections in humans. The risk of burn in females is more than that of a male because women can use cooking stoves or open cooking fires daily. While in males the risk of burn is less but it is present as in the form of alcoholism and smoking which is common in males. Burn occurs as a result of violence or self-harm. In the USA the common causes of burn are given as burn from the chemical is 3%, burn from electricity is 4%, burns due to scalding are 33%, burn from fire is 44%. Most of the injuries caused by the burn which 69% is at home. 2% assaulted burn injuries can be reported in the USA [1]. 1-2% burn injuries reported due to the suicide attempt which comes in the category of self-harm [2].

[*] **Corresponding author Muhammad Imran Qadir:** Institute of Molecular Biology and Biotechnology, Bahauddin Zakariya University, Multan, Pakistan; Tel: +92-61-9210071; Ext. 1920; Fax: +92-61-9210068; E-mail: mrimranqadir@hotmail.com

Muhammad Imran Qadir (Ed.)
All rights reserved-© 2020 Bentham Science Publishers

Smoking causes 25% of burns in the USA or heating device here causes a 22% burn. The electrical burn causes a 60% burn in children.

SYMPTOMS AND TYPES

There are three types of burns. It exists upon which layer of your skin can be damaged by burn either it can be epidermis (the outer layer of skin), dermis (layer of tissue just beneath the skin), subcutis (deeper layer containing fat or tissue) superficial epidermal burn (epidermis is damage) or dermal burn epidermis or part of dermis damage), Partial-thickness burns (dermis and epidermis damaged), full-thickness burn all three layers of skin damaged epidermis, dermis or subcutis. Burn causes bacterial infection or increases the risk of sepsis. Burns damage blood vessels making low blood volume. Burn some time happens to cause breathing problems due to the smoke of the fire. Burn causes bone or joint problems due to the shortening or tightening of skin or muscle tendons. Burns causes the skin to be red, pale pink, dry blotchy, moist, swollen, and blistered, the texture of the skin can be leathery or waxy, brown or black with no blisters.

TREATMENT

Take away the person from the heat source. Immediately cool down the burn area with lukewarm water, ice water can note be used. Remove the greasy substances from the burn area. Remove the clothes or the jewelry from the burnt area of skin. Use a blanket to make the body warm but not rub that area of the body by using cling films to cover the area of the burn. For hand, burns plastic bags can be used. If the face or eye area is burnt then, to reduce swelling, a person should sit up instead of lying down.

PREVENTION

Keep the children away from the kitchen. Keep children away from hot drinks. Handle electrical appliances or instruments with CARE. Use chemicals with his/her proper care. Matches lighters or candles should be out of the reach of children.

DIAGNOSIS

Burn can be diagnosed by examination. First, we check its source either it is heat burn or chemical burn. Then we check its depth on how deep it is and see how much area is affected. Burn depth can be examined through biopsy. It can be difficult to find the accurate depth of a burn. In the case of the fire-related burn which causes "dizziness or headache," these are symptoms that can be treated by carbon monoxide poisoning or cyanide poisoning. Estimation of the damaged part of burn can be done by Lund or Browder charts which account for or perform various proportions of body parts determine. It can be divided into the minor, major moderate burn. Minor burn treated at home. Moderate burn treated at hospitals. Major burn treated in a burn center Fig. (**5**).

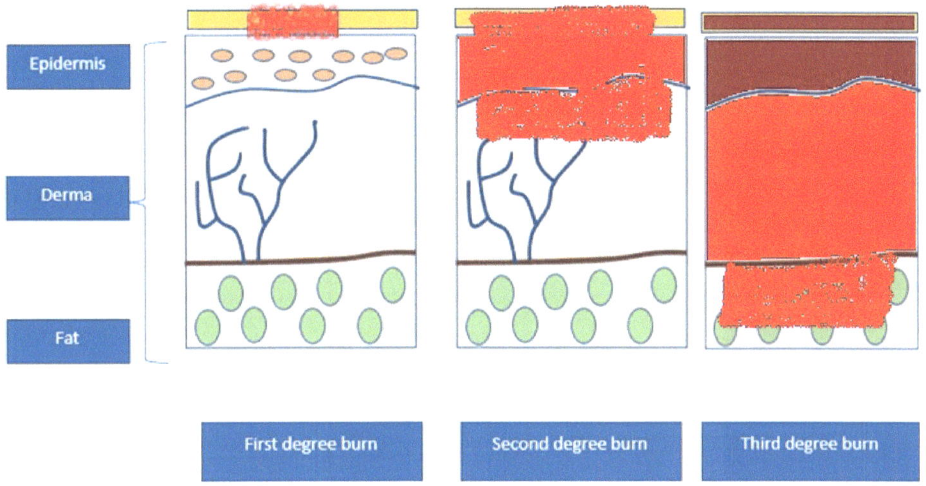

Fig. (5). Degree of burns.

MANAGEMENT

Treated patient with stabilization of airway, circulation, and breathing. Intubation is necessary if inhalation injury is expected and is followed by self-care of the burn wound. Treatment of burn wounds can be through medication surgery and self-care.

Medication

Medication can be through intravenous and oral. Analgesics can be used such as acetaminophen and also opioids can be used to treat burns patients like morphine. Burns are painful sometimes different pain killers were given to relieve the pain.

Surgery

We can do surgery to immediately treat a burn scar. We can do escharotomy to treat the skin of limbs or chest. In the case of electrical burns, fasciotomies can be required.

Traditional Treatments

We can use honey from ancient times to treat the severity of burns. Aloe Vera can be used to relieve the pain of burns although it cannot be as efficient as honey sometimes it can prove to be beneficial to improve healing [3]. Some researchers said that vitamin E can be helpful in scar treatment [4]. Underdeveloped countries can mostly use traditional methods to treat burn infection due to poor income. They can use mud, cow manure, "egg" and sometimes leaves can be used.

CONSENT FOR PUBLICATION

Not applicable.

CONFLICT OF INTEREST

The authors declare no conflict of interest, financial or otherwise.

ACKNOWLEDGEMENTS

Declared none.

REFERENCES

[1]   Peck MD. Epidemiology of burns throughout the world. Part I: Distribution and risk factors. Burns 2011; 37(7): 1087-100.
[http://dx.doi.org/10.1016/j.burns.2011.06.005] [PMID: 21802856]

[2]   WOLF SE. CANCIO LC, PRUITT B Epidemiological, Demographic and Outcome Characteristics of Burns. Total Burn Care E-Book 2017; p. 314.

[3]   Dat AD, Poon F, Pham KB, Doust J. Aloe vera for treating acute and chronic wounds. Cochrane Database Syst Rev 2012; (2): CD008762.
[http://dx.doi.org/10.1002/14651858.CD008762.pub2] [PMID: 22336851]

[4]   Juckett G, Hartman-Adams H. Management of keloids and hypertrophic scars. Am Fam Physician 2009; 80(3): 253-60.
[PMID: 19621835]

CHAPTER 9

Gas Gangrene: *Clostridial Myonecrosis*

Muhammad Imran Qadir[*] and **Hafiza Sobia Khan**

Institute of Molecular Biology & Biotechnology, Bahauddin Zakariya University, Multan, Pakistan

Abstract: Gas gangrene is a life-threatening disease which is caused by anaerobic bacteria. Most commonly the infection is a result of any kind of injury or wound. Bacteria grow in the wounded area when an individual does not take care of his wound. Different tests are available for the diagnosis of gangrene infection including a blood test or imaging tests. Treatment can be possible either through antibiotics or surgery. Hyperbaric oxygen therapy considered a lifesaving therapy as it increases the survival rate. Prevention is better in case of infection rather than cure after infection.

Keywords: Anaerobic Bacteria, Gangrene, Infection.

INTRODUCTION

Gas gangrene another term used for *clostridial myonecrosis* caused by a bacteria *Clostridium* perfringens. C. perfringens is an aerobic, spore-forming gram-positive bacteria that resides in the intestine of humans as well as in animals, but is commonly found in soil [1]. Myonecrosis is a state of tissue damage while gangrene means dead tissues. During the infection, a gas is produced in these dead or damaged tissues. Gas gangrene is divided into three main categories; post-traumatic, post-operative, and spontaneous type [2]. The third one that is a spontaneous type that is caused by *C. perfringens* has a high mortality rate [3]. The spontaneous myonecrosis mostly occurs in patients of diabetes [4]. Not only *Clostridium* perfringens cause myonecrosis infection but also there are certain other strains of bacteria like *Clostridium* septicum, *Clostridium* novyi, *Clostridium* bifermentans, *Clostridium* fallax, and *Clostridium* histolyticum. Among these *C. perfringens*, *C. navy* and *C. septicum* infections are most common [5].

---

[*] **Corresponding author Muhammad Imran Qadir:** Institute of Molecular Biology and Biotechnology, Bahauddin Zakariya University, Multan, Pakistan; Tel: +92-61-9210071; Ext. 1920; Fax: +92-61-9210068; E-mail: mrimranqadir@hotmail.com

Muhammad Imran Qadir (Ed.)
All rights reserved-© 2020 Bentham Science Publishers

CAUSES OF GAS GANGRENE

Some of the main causes of gas gangrene are as follows;

A Limited Supply of Blood

Sometimes due to clogged, shrunk, or restricted blood vessels, blood cannot reach the specific tissues and the result is tissue damage at that particular site. This is one of the major causes of this infection.

Trauma

Tissue damage due to wounds or injuries that are a result of serious injuries like severe accident or gunshot. Sometimes bacteria raid in the tissues and cause infection which turns to myonecrosis.

Infection

When bacteria successfully colonize at a specific part or tissue they start damaging tissues and the ultimate result is infection.

Some other factors which contribute to infection are excessive use of tobacco, obesity, use of illegal drugs, immunosuppression, and also some diseases like diabetes and liver cirrhosis.

PREVENTION

Some of the measures can help in the prevention of infection and these are:

- Take care of your diabetes and examine your hands and feet regularly.
- Prevent smoking.
- Control your obesity.
- In case of wounds try to keep them clean.

PREVALENCE

The mortality rate of myonecrosis infection is about 20-30% but it can be increased up to 50-80% depending on how much infection spreads.

DIAGNOSIS

Early diagnosis of the infection is a very difficult task. Early signs of *C. perfringens* infection include sudden changes in a wound, fever, and accumulation of fluid under the skin or wound area, and sometimes changes in mental health conditions [6].

Blood Test

If the level of WBCs in the blood is elevated abnormally then there are chances of the presence of these bacteria.

Surgery

Surgery of the infection determines how much infection spreads in the body of the patient.

Tissue Culturing

Fluids or tissues are taken from the site of infection as a sample and culture in the labs to see the presence of bacteria.

Imaging Test

Certain imaging tests like MRI, CT-scan, and X-rays can also be used to see the presence of gas in the tissues.

MANAGEMENT

Damaged tissues cannot be saved, but some measurements can be used to treat the disease, and doctors suggest one of these depending on the extent of infection.

Surgery

During the surgery, dead tissues are removed to prevent the spread of infection. More than one surgeries re-performed.

Antibiotics

Intravenous or oral antibiotics are given. Penicillin most commonly used in *C. perfringens* infection [7].

Hyperbaric Oxygen Therapy

Besides surgery and antibiotics, hyperbaric oxygen therapy can also be performed to treat gangrene infection. This therapy reduces the mortality rate [8]. During this therapy the patient is situated in a camber; especially design for this and pasteurized with pure oxygen. The treatment lasts for about 60-90 minutes and the patient needs about 2-3 treatments daily.

CONSENT FOR PUBLICATION

Not applicable.

CONFLICT OF INTEREST

The authors declare no conflict of interest, financial or otherwise.

ACKNOWLEDGEMENTS

Declared none.

REFERENCES

[1]   Stevens DL, Bryant AE. The role of clostridial toxins in the pathogenesis of gas gangrene 2002.
        [http://dx.doi.org/10.1086/341928]

[2]   Kuroda S, Okada Y, Mita M, *et al.* Fulminant massive gas gangrene caused by *Clostridium perfringens*. Intern Med 2005; 44(5): 499-502.
        [http://dx.doi.org/10.2169/internalmedicine.44.499] [PMID: 15942103]

[3]   Lamb R, Hart G, Strauss M. Gas gangrene: a collective review. J Trauma 1983; 23: 991-5.
        [http://dx.doi.org/10.1097/00005373-198311000-00006]

[4]   Chen Y-M, Lee H-C, Chang C-M, Chuang Y-C, Ko W-C. Clostridium bacteremia: emphasis on the poor prognosis in cirrhotic patients 2001.

[5]   MacLennan JD. The histotoxic clostridial infections of man. Bacteriol Rev 1962; 26(2 Pt 1-2): 177-276.
        [http://dx.doi.org/10.1128/MMBR.26.2_Pt_1-2.177-274.1962] [PMID: 14468017]

[6]   Hart G, Strauss M. Gas gangrene-*clostridial myonecrosis*: A review 1990.

[7]   Altemeier WA, Fullen WD. Prevention and treatment of gas gangrene. JAMA 1971; 217(6): 806-13.
        [http://dx.doi.org/10.1001/jama.1971.03190060046011] [PMID: 5109333]

[8]   Jackson RW, Waddell JP. Hyperbaric oxygen in the management of *clostridial myonecrosis* (gas gangrene). Clin Orthop Relat Res 1973; (96): 271-6.
        [http://dx.doi.org/10.1097/00003086-197310000-00037] [PMID: 4749823]

CHAPTER 10

Spontaneous Bacterial Peritonitis: Accumulation of Fluids in the Abdomen in Abnormal Way

Muhammad Imran Qadir[*] and **Sadia Ishfaq**

Institute of Molecular Biology & Biotechnology, Bahauddin Zakariya University, Multan, Pakistan

Abstract: Spontaneous bacterial peritonitis is a disease that is associated with other types of disorders. It occurs due to the storage of fluids in the abdomen in an abnormal way as well as in the absence of abscess such as intra-abdominal inflammatory focus. Various types of bacteria are involved in this infection these may be both aerobic and anaerobic as well as gram-negative and gram-positive bacteria *e.g.* klebsiella, pneumonia, and some species of streptococcus pneumonia. People suffering from heart diseases and liver disorders have more chances of this disease. About 20% of the patients die due to this disease.

Keywords: Klebsiella, Pneumonia.

INTRODUCTION

Spontaneous bacterial peritonitis also abbreviated as (SBP) can be defined as a severe infection of ascites that is the accumulation of fluids in the abdomen in an abnormal way. The most obvious cause of SBP is anaerobic gram-negative bacteria of which 50% species were of Klebsiella pneumoniae. 75%of SBP is caused by gram-negative bacteria and 25% are caused by gram-positive bacteria including Streptococcus pneumoniae or viridans. SBP occurs in children as well as in adults mostly in the children of 5 years old [1]. Chances of this disease become more obvious in the patients who suffered from cirrhosis (a disease in which liver cannot work properly because of long-term disturbance of liver as normal liver tissues are replaced with the scar tissues) it can also occur as a complication of any disorder that causes accumulation of ascitic fluid these disorders are liver disease, budd- chiari syndrome, congestive heart failure, renal failure, and cancer. About 10% to 25% of the people having such disorders have more chances of SBP of which 20% have the chances of death. It can also occur

[*] **Corresponding author Muhammad Imran Qadir:** Institute of Molecular Biology and Biotechnology, Bahauddin Zakariya University, Multan, Pakistan; Tel: +92-61-9210071; Ext. 1920; Fax: +92-61-9210068; E-mail: mrimranqadir@hotmail.com

Muhammad Imran Qadir (Ed.)
All rights reserved-© 2020 Bentham Science Publishers

due to the absence of visceral perforation and intra-abdominal inflammatory focus *e.g.* abscess.

SYMPTOMS

Patients suffering from SBP have a severe history of medical deterioration. Major symptoms of SBP that occur in the majority of patients are chills, abdominal pain fever, diarrhea, paralytic ileus, and changed mental status (new-onset encephalopathy). On examination, some patients also have tender abdomen [2]. The most common symptom is a fever that proves as a clinically beneficial symptom as the temperature of the body increases in the condition of cirrhosis. In some cases, SBP may occur without any symptoms and can be incidentally found.

Most of the patients suffer from fever which is the most obvious symptom of spontaneous bacterial peritonitis. Thus patients can be easily identified.

CAUSES

Some causes of spontaneous bacterial peritonitis are various types of disorders related to heart, brain, kidney increase in the number of poly morpho-nuclear leukocytes (PML). If these PML increases more than 250 cells/μ the risk factor increases by up to 93%.

BACTERIAL TRANSLOCATION

In some cases, SBP results due to translocation of bacteria from the gut which increases the risk of changes in the gut flora and also causes resistance in the functions of gut flora. This increases the risk factors of SBP. It is also stated that these bacteria cause SBP to come from the intestinal lumen.

Some other causes of SBP:

- Heart disorders
- Kidney failure
- Cirrhosis
- Cancer
- Budd chiari syndrome.

People suffering from these diseases have more chances of SBP.

MANAGEMENT AND CONTROL

The fluid of the peritoneum is analyzed by counting the cells, by checking the lactate level, by measuring pH level. All the patients who are suspected of SBP should be examined properly this can also be treated by removal of the fluid from the peritoneum by using catheters. Ultrasonography is also used in patients who have mild effects of SBP. Cultures of blood and urine are also collected from the patients who determine the infection site. All these measures should be taken before starting antibiotic therapy.

Some cirrhotic patients with SBP and either a serum creatinine greater than 1mg/dL, a blood urea nitrogen (BUN) greater than 30mg/dL, or total bilirubin greater than 4mg/dL should be given adjunctive (*i.e.* , in addition to antibiotics) albumin intravenously. This has been shown to reduce both in-hospital mortality and renal damage when compared to the use of antibiotic therapy alone.

CONSENT FOR PUBLICATION

Not applicable.

CONFLICT OF INTEREST

The authors declare no conflict of interest, financial or otherwise.

ACKNOWLEDGEMENTS

Declared none.

REFERENCES

[1]   Mazzaferro V, Regalia E, Doci R, *et al.* Liver transplantation for the treatment of small hepatocellular carcinomas in patients with cirrhosis. N Engl J Med 1996; 334(11): 693-9.
[http://dx.doi.org/10.1056/NEJM199603143341104] [PMID: 8594428]

[2]   Such J, Runyon BA. Spontaneous bacterial peritonitis. Clin Infect Dis 1998; 27(4): 669-74.
[http://dx.doi.org/10.1086/514940] [PMID: 9798013]

CHAPTER 11

Relapsing Fever: Transmitted by Ticks and Lice

Muhammad Imran Qadir[*] and **Rimshah Khan**
Institute of Molecular Biology & Biotechnology, Bahauddin Zakariya University, Multan, Pakistan

Abstract: Relapsing fever has been a major epidemic disease in Europe and Africa. It is transmitted by tick or louse and has two types, LBRF and TBRF. Patients have repeated episodes of fever and other symptoms. The cause of infection is Borrelia species of bacteria. It is treated by antibiotics and single doses are preferred over multiple doses because multiple doses are difficult to implement.

Keywords: Borrelia Species, Control, Episodes of Fever, Treatment, Types of Relapsing Fevers.

INTRODUCTION

Relapsing fever has been one of the major epidemic diseases because of its significant impact on Livingstone throughout Europe and Africa. The clinical cases of this disease were first used to describe in Edinburgh. It is a kind of infection transmitted by louse or tick. The patient has recurring fever episodes and other nonspecific symptoms *e.g.* headaches, joint aches, muscle aches, nausea, stiff neck, shaking chills, seizure, and coma. The infection caused by borrelia species causes the illness. The Borrelia species have different surface antigens leading to repeated spirochaetosis and thus the immune system is stimulated by each new antigen and the febrile response is given by the patient [1].

TYPES AND CAUSES OF RELAPSING FEVER

There are two types of relapsing fever.

- TBRF (tick-borne relapsing fever) it is transmitted by *Ornithodoros tick*. These are the bacterial species that causes the TBRF is *Borrelia duttoni*, *Borrelia hermsii*, *Borrelia parkerii*. This kind of relapsing fever usually occurs in Spain, Asia, Saudi Arabia, and in some specific areas of the United States.

---

[*] **Corresponding author Muhammad Imran Qadir:** Institute of Molecular Biology and Biotechnology, Bahauddin Zakariya University, Multan, Pakistan; Tel: +92 61 9210071; Ext. 1920, Fax. 92-61-9210068; E-mail: mrimranqadir@hotmail.com

Muhammad Imran Qadir (Ed.)
All rights reserved-© 2020 Bentham Science Publishers

- LBRF (louse-borne relapsing fever) is transferred from body lice and is associated with *Borrelia recurrentis*. This disease is present in Asia, Africa, and South America. Now by improving the living standards of a human being caused a reduction of body lice which is the vector for *Borrelia recurrentis* (louse-borne relapsing fever) [2]. The tick-borne relapsing fever is caused by spirochete *Borrelia crocidura*. This pathogen is transferred by the tick *Ornithodoros sonrai* formerly *Alectorobius sonrai*. This tick is an ectoparasite, it used to live in insectivores and rodents.

EFFECTS AND SYMPTOMS

This disease affects people during their sleep because the hosts make burrows in the bedrooms. This disease can cause illness in people. If this disease is not treated people could have this fever for months and many complications of severe meningoencephalitis can occur [3]. In tick-borne relapsing fever, the patient has recurring episodes of fever which may last up to 3 days. Then the patient does not have the fever up to 2 weeks, and then it returns. In louse-borne relapsing fever, the fever occurs and remains for 3 to 6 days this is usually the only and milder episode of fever. The fever in both forms of relapsing fever ends in trouble. This can be fatal and can lead to death when there are shaking chills, low blood pressure, sweating, and falling body temperature. Relapsing fever is usually the infection of blood but it can also affect the eyes and nervous system. After clinical examinations and treatments of relapsing fever of humans, the results showed that *Borrelia turicatae* and *Borrelia duttonii* which are the agents of tick-borne relapsing fever can cause involvement in the nervous system. Lymphocytic meningitis and facial palsy frequent occurrence in the brain and other tissues of the nervous system of humans and the brain infections persistence even after treatment with antibiotics that do not penetrate the blood-brain barrier, it proves the above logic [4].

TREATMENT

Antibiotics are used for the treatment of relapsing fevers. The single dose of antibiotics is preferred over multiple doses which are difficult to implement. Antibiotics that can be used for treatment could be penicillin, tetracyclines, ampicillin, and erythromycin [5]. In adults, patients having louse-borne relapsing fever single dose of tetracycline 500 mg, while doxycycline 200 mg is given. In case if tetracyclines are in counter position than 500 mg erythromycin is given.

POSSIBILITY OF CONTROL

The relapsing fever has been reducing from global infection to a very small region so it might lead to speculation that we could eradicate this disease. For this, we need to understand the interactions of spirochete with its host and vectors. It can be possible that spirochete is adapted to transmission of a louse from tick-borne *B. duttonii,* it can also be possible that ticks are the reason for the transfer of *B. recurrentis.* The cloth lice are eliminated significantly but the headlice is still present. Headlice is still a major problem worldwide. The ability of these spirochetes to persevere within immunologically protected niches *e.g.* brain could serve as a source for revival of infection [6].

CONSENT FOR PUBLICATION

Not applicable.

CONFLICT OF INTEREST

The authors declare no conflict of interest, financial or otherwise.

ACKNOWLEDGEMENTS

Declared none.

REFERENCES

[1]   Dworkin MS, Schwan TG, Anderson DE Jr, Borchardt SM. Tick-borne relapsing fever. Infect Dis Clin North Am 2008; 22(3): 449-468, viii.
        [http://dx.doi.org/10.1016/j.idc.2008.03.006] [PMID: 18755384]

[2]   Cutler SJ. Relapsing fever--a forgotten disease revealed. J Appl Microbiol 2010; 108(4): 1115-22.
        [http://dx.doi.org/10.1111/j.1365-2672.2009.04598.x] [PMID: 19886891]

[3]   Vial L, Diatta G, Tall A, *et al.* Incidence of tick-borne relapsing fever in west Africa: longitudinal study. Lancet 2006; 368(9529): 37-43.
        [http://dx.doi.org/10.1016/S0140-6736(06)68968-X] [PMID: 16815378]

[4]   Cadavid D, Barbour AG. Neuroborreliosis during relapsing fever: review of the clinical manifestations, pathology, and treatment of infections in humans and experimental animals. Clin Infect Dis 1998; 26(1): 151-64.
        [http://dx.doi.org/10.1086/516276] [PMID: 9455525]

[5]   Goubau PF. Relapsing fevers. A review. Ann Soc Belg Med Trop 1984; 64(4): 335-64.
        [PMID: 6397148]

[6]   Radolf JD, Samuels DS. Borrelia: molecular biology, host interaction, and pathogenesis. Horizon Scientific Press 2010.

CHAPTER 12

Rat-bite Fever: *Streptobacillus Moniliformis* and *Spirillum Minus* Infection

Muhammad Imran Qadir[*] and **Rameen Fatima**

Institute of Molecular Biology & Biotechnology, Bahauddin Zakariya University, Multan, Pakistan

Abstract: Rat-bite fever is a zoonotic infection that is caused by these two bacteria *Streptobacillus moniliformis* and *Spirillum minus*. These two bacteria cause similar but distinct infections, that are transmitted through rats bite, mucous or other feces. It is a rare disease and practices are uncommon on this infection it can be fatal if not treated on time. It is transmitted through rat's feces, mucous of rat mouth, nose or may be transmitted through contaminated products with rats. Patients undergo fever, rashes, joint pain due to infection. Moniliform bacteria cause Arthritis. As, there is no vaccine available for Rat-bite fever, practices on development for infection treatment are on the way. Antibiotics and Antiallergens are available to cure rashes and infection. This infection can cause syndromes, so treatment on time and preventive measurement are necessary.

Keywords: Human Infections, Rat-Bite Fever, *Streptobacillus moniliformis*, *Spirillum minus*.

INTRODUCTION

It is a disease caused by two bacteria *Streptobacillus moniliformis* and *Spirillum minus* transmitted by rats. Humans infected with this disease through rats. It can be transmitted through food that humans eat and contaminated with infectious rat secretions from mouth, eyes, and nose. Other animals that are exposed to contaminated things or infectious mucous may be disease transfer to humans. Other carriers of this disease are pet animals such as cats and dogs that can infect humans when exposed to infectious rats [1].

But this disease is more spread by the bite of a rat than other contaminated things. In history, this disease attacked only lab-workers that do experiments on rats by a bite or to peoples who are living miserable lifestyle. But, over time when people

[*] **Corresponding author Muhammad Imran Qadir:** Institute of Molecular Biology and Biotechnology, Bahauddin Zakariya University, Multan, Pakistan; Tel: +92-61-9210071; Ext. 1920; Fax: +92-61-9210068; E-mail: mrimranqadir@hotmail.com

Muhammad Imran Qadir (Ed.)
All rights reserved-© 2020 Bentham Science Publishers

take rat as pet animal rats start attacking children and they get infected more by this disease [2].

It has different alternative names such as epidemic arthritic erythema, streptobacillary, spirally fever based on its symptoms, or bacteria that infect. In Asia infection is more spread by *Spirillum minus*. If proper treatment is not done, it will cause a 13% mortality rate. 1% of bites are by rats Each year 2 million peoples infected with infectious diseases and 1% is with rats bite. Wild and Pet rats are both causes infection by biting mostly in children's and workers that work in pet houses and labs. In some cases, it would be cured in a year, but it might take a longer time to end or maybe a death in some infections [3].

These bacteria that cause infection are anaerobic, facultative, and gram-negative bacteria. These two bacteria cause different two diseases that are distinct.

STREPTOBACILLOSIS

It causes Haverhill fever and arthritic erythema by moniliforms bacteria. After two to ten days this fever start showing other symptoms such as pain in joints, cold, pain in the head, and cause death if not treated on time. In 20% of cases, it will cause death, if left untreated.

SPIRILLOSIS

It is also known as sodoku. Symptoms do not appear in **2-4** weeks of infection. Gastrointestinal, rectal pain is not severe in this bacterial infection but fever lasts for a long time than it cures. It is mostly found in the Asian region [4].

SYMPTOMS

Its symptoms vary with the type of bacteria which infect a person with different strains. Some of the symptoms are common in every infected person, but some are specific types of every individual bacterial infection. These symptoms come in different phases during wound healing. In 2-10 days after infection generally, symptoms start appears. Peoples living in poor sanitary conditions are at risk of this disease, as have more risk of bitten through rats [5].

- Rashes on the infection area, the colour becomes purple or reddish.
- Aches in muscles of an infected person.
- Swallowed and painful joints of an infected person.
- Inflammation on skin and itching due to infection [6].
- The swelling of lymph nodes, particularly in the underarm or in the neck.
- It leads to fever, rashes, tenderness, and pain in joints [7].

DIAGNOSIS

There are different tests present for testing different strains. Such as;

- Blood Antibody Tests
- Direct visualization
    - In the diagnosis of *S. minus* bacteria, Direct Visualization is done of samples taken from lymph nodes, tissue, or maybe blood.
    - In the diagnosis of Moniliforms bacteria, fluid taken from joints is cultured having organisms [8].

PREVENTIVE MEASURES

By taking preventive measures, the risk factor for this disease can be decreased, as there is no vaccine generated for this infectious disease [9].

- Wash hands after touching rats or any animal that can become a vector of that infectious disease.
- Take care of pets and be sure not to ingest those animals with infection.
- Antiseptics should be used after working with those animals in labs, pet houses by care-takers, or laboratory workers [10].

MANAGEMENT

If not treated, it will cause some infections of disease to cause deaths. It affects the lungs, brain, spinal; cord, and heart inner-lining [11].

- Spirillosis which is also known as sudoku treated by Antibiotic Penicillin.
- Streptobacillosis which is treated by Penicillin or maybe by Doxycycline or Tetracycline.
    - Antibiotic is the only option for the treatment of rat-bite fever because there is no prepared vaccine for the disease. Erythromycin is used for allergic reactions with Rat-bite fever [12].

CONCLUSION

Rat-Bite Fever is characterized as rashes or inflammation on the skin. It is a bacterial disease transmitted by rats to humans. It is an infectious disease and causes other types of diseases, such as fever, headache, joints pain, and inflammation, or rashes on an infected or bitten place on the skin. Antibiotics are used to cure it. But, preventive measures and awareness about this infection can help people to save from rat bites and rat-bite fever.

CONSENT FOR PUBLICATION

Not applicable.

CONFLICT OF INTEREST

The authors declare no conflict of interest, financial or otherwise.

ACKNOWLEDGEMENTS

Declared none.

REFERENCES

[1]   Walker JW, Reyes LB. Rat Bite Fever: A Case Report and Review of the Literature. Pediatr Emerg Care 2016.
        [PMID: 28002119]

[2]   Elliott SP. Rat bite fever and *Streptobacillus moniliformis*. Clin Microbiol Rev 2007; 20(1): 13-22.
        [http://dx.doi.org/10.1128/CMR.00016-06] [PMID: 17223620]

[3]   Gaastra W, Boot R, Ho HT, Lipman LJ. Rat bite fever. Vet Microbiol 2009; 133(3): 211-28.
        [http://dx.doi.org/10.1016/j.vetmic.2008.09.079] [PMID: 19008054]

[4]   Fatal rat-bite fever--Florida and Washington, 2003. MMWR Morb Mortal Wkly Rep 2005; 53(51): 1198-202.
        [PMID: 15635289]

[5]   Rahman S, Adegboyega A, Rowland K. Fever, petechiae, and joint pain. J Fam Pract 2017; 66(5): 323-5.
        [PMID: 28459894]

[6]   Rahman S, Adegboyega A, Rowland K. Fever, petechiae, and joint pain. J Fam Pract 2017; 66(5): 323-5.
        [PMID: 28459894]

[7]   Graves MH, Janda JM. Rat-bite fever (*Streptobacillus moniliformis*): a potential emerging disease. Int J Infect Dis 2001; 5(3): 151-5.
        [http://dx.doi.org/10.1016/S1201-9712(01)90090-6] [PMID: 11724672]

[8]   Eisenberg T, Poignant S, Jouan Y, *et al.* Acute Tetraplegia Caused by Rat Bite Fever in Snake Keeper and Transmission of *Streptobacillus moniliformis*. Emerg Infect Dis 2017; 23(4): 719-21.
        [http://dx.doi.org/10.3201/eid2304.161987] [PMID: 28322713]

[9]   Damborg P, Broens EM, Chomel BB, *et al.* Bacterial zoonoses transmitted by household pets: State of the art and future perspectives for targeted research and policy actions. J Comp Pathol 2016; 155(1) (Suppl. 1): S27-40.
        [http://dx.doi.org/10.1016/j.jcpa.2015.03.004] [PMID: 25958184]

[10]   Baddour L, Harper M, Wiley JF. Patient education: animal and human bites (beyond the basics). 2017.

[11]   Stull JW, Brophy J, Weese JS. Reducing the risk of pet-associated zoonotic infections. CMAJ 2015; 187(10): 736-43.
        [http://dx.doi.org/10.1503/cmaj.141020] [PMID: 25897046]

[12]   Rosser A, Wiselka M, Pareek M. Rat bite fever: an unusual cause of a maculopapular rash. Postgrad Med J 2014; 90(1062): 236-7.
        [http://dx.doi.org/10.1136/postgradmedj-2013-132420] [PMID: 24453224]

CHAPTER 13

Brucellosis: A *Brucella* Infection

Muhammad Imran Qadir[*] and **Nadia Wazir**

Institute of Molecular Biology & Biotechnology, Bahauddin Zakariya University, Multan, Pakistan

Abstract: Brucellosis is a bacterial disease that affects humans and cattle. In humans, Brucellosis is characterized by nonspecific influenza and fever-like symptoms. Brucellosis is caused by different strains of *Brucella* like *B. abortus, B. melitensis, B. suis, and B. canis*. Brucellosis is transferred from sexual contact or breastfeeding. Brucella infection is rare without contact with tissue or blood. Proper treatment of this disease not done timely then it becomes a chronic and life-threatening but very rare case it may cause death. Brucellosis in humans is transmitted through animals. Eating of raw animal products may have a high risk of brucellosis these products are raw meat and unpasteurized milk products. Testing may include are Urine culture, Blood culture, Bone marrow, Testing for antibodies, and Cerebrospinal fluid testing. Avoid consuming raw materials of animals like cheese, ice-cream, unpasteurized milk, and meat.

Keywords: Brucellosis, *Brucella* Species of Bacteria, Risk Factors, Infection.

INTRODUCTION

Brucellosis is a zoonoses disease. It can affect any organ of the body, but the most important infection is gastrointestinal. Brucellosis is a systematic infection or Malta fever that considers myalgias, arthralgias, and sweats. Brucellosis is a disease caused by a group of bacteria from the same genus known as *Brucella*. This type of bacteria causes infection in both humans and animals [1]. Brucellosis is spread due to the eating of contaminated food in which include raw meat and unpasteurized milk. This bacterium is transferred due to air or contact with an open wound [2].

RISK FACTORS THAT EFFECTS THE DISEASE

Brucella bacteria are present in saliva and animal vault. Different animals contract with brucelloses like goats, cows, and dogs. Brucellosis is transferred in humans

---

[*] **Corresponding author Muhammad Imran Qadir:** Institute of Molecular Biology and Biotechnology, Bahauddin Zakariya University, Multan, Pakistan; Tel: +92-61-9210071; Ext. 1920; Fax: +92-61-9210068; E-mail: mrimranqadir@hotmail.com

Muhammad Imran Qadir (Ed.)
All rights reserved-© 2020 Bentham Science Publishers

by contact with infected animals. Different Bacteria of *Brucella* species are *B. abortus, B. melitensis, B. suis, and B. canis* can transfer through contact with open a wound, ingestion, and inhaling. In these cases, if you spent more time in animals [3]. Brucellosis is easily transferred from an animal to humans. The risk of brucellosis is higher in those people who contact with animal blood, tissue, and urine. Sometimes, Brucellosis is transferred in casual contact with animals. Eating of raw animal products may have a high risk of brucellosis [4]. The products that carry *Brucella* bacteria are raw meat and unpasteurized milk and cheese. The chance of getting brucellosis is higher when you eating affected meat and raw dairy products from the area of Europe, Asia, and Africa where the disease is more common in the world [5].

SYMPTOMS

The followings are the symptoms of brucellosis in humans are similar to like flu that may include Headaches, Lethargy, Chills, Back pain, Loss of appetite, Pain in bone and joint, pain in the abdomen, loss of weight and Fever that comes and goes.

TRANSMISSION OF DISEASE

Brucellosis is rarely transferring from one human to another. Brucellosis is transferred from sexual contact or breastfeeding. Infection of this is rare without contact with tissue or blood.

DIAGNOSIS OF BRUCELLOSIS

Testing may include are Urine culture, Blood culture, Bone marrow, Testing for antibodies, and Cerebrospinal fluid testing. Doctors may test you, when you have not explained flu-like symptoms and contact with animals then the above tests are recommended that might have brucellosis [6]. Exposures of Brucellosis are not recent even sometimes months or years ago to contact with animals [7].

TREATMENT

Treatment of Brucellosis takes at least six weeks. Doctors may prescribe antibiotics like Doxycycline and rifampin.

Complications of Brucellosts

Sometimes antibiotics will not kill brucella bacteria. Doctors may prescribe some other drugs to treat this disease. Brucellosis causes complications, in that case, their treatment is not successful. These may include:

- Endocarditis (Infection of heart inner lining)
- Lesion on the bones and joints
- Encephalitis and meningitis (inflammation of the brain and membrane around your brain)
- Anorexia
- Depression

Some complications are lethal, but death from brucellosis is rare [8]. The mortality rate is less than two percent from brucellosis. Most cases of this disease can survive if they do not have any complications [9].

Prevention Measures of Brucellosis

Lower chances of brucellosis, you should have to vaccinate by brucellosis. Unfortunately, there is no vaccine is available, that's why following the steps are important to protect yourself from brucellosis:

- Always wears gloves and protective glasses when handling animal tissues and animals.
- Cover your skin and open wound when you contact with animal blood.
- Always wear protective gloves and clothing when helping in animal birth.
- Avoid consuming raw materials of animals like cheese, ice-cream, unpasteurized milk, and meat.

To lower the chance of getting brucellosis, it is preventable [6].

CONSENT FOR PUBLICATION

Not applicable.

CONFLICT OF INTEREST

The authors declare no conflict of interest, financial or otherwise.

ACKNOWLEDGEMENTS

Declared none.

REFERENCES

[1]   Holmes J. Diversity and change in Australia's rangelands: a post–productivist transition with a difference? Trans Inst Br Geogr 2002; 27(3): 362-84.
[http://dx.doi.org/10.1111/1475-5661.00059]

[2]   Russell-Lodrigue KE, Killeen SZ, Ficht TA, Roy CJ. Mucosal bacterial dissemination in a rhesus macaque model of experimental brucellosis. J Med Primatol 2018; 47(1): 75-7.

[http://dx.doi.org/10.1111/jmp.12282] [PMID: 28573738]

[3]   Abdelbaset AE, Abushahba MFN, Hamed MI, Rawy MS. Sero-diagnosis of brucellosis in sheep and humans in Assiut and El-Minya governorates, Egypt. Int J Vet Sci Med 2018; 6 (Suppl.): S63-7.
[http://dx.doi.org/10.1016/j.ijvsm.2018.01.007] [PMID: 30761323]

[4]   Mor SM, Wiethoelter AK, Massey PD, Robson J, Wilks K, Hutchinson P. Pigs, pooches and pasteurisation: The changing face of brucellosis in Australia. Aust J Gen Pract 2018; 47(3): 99-103.
[http://dx.doi.org/10.31128/AFP-08-17-4289] [PMID: 29621840]

[5]   Cossaboom CM, Kharod GA, Salzer JS, *et al.* Notes from the Field: *Brucella abortus* Vaccine Strain RB51 Infection and Exposures Associated with Raw Milk Consumption - Wise County, Texas, 2017. MMWR Morb Mortal Wkly Rep 2018; 67(9): 286.
[http://dx.doi.org/10.15585/mmwr.mm6709a4] [PMID: 29518066]

[6]   Krkić-Dautović S, Mehanić S, Ferhatović M, Čavaljuga S. Brucellosis epidemiological and clinical aspects (Is brucellosis a major public health problem in Bosnia and Herzegovina?). Bosn J Basic Med Sci 2006; 6(2): 11-5.
[PMID: 16879106]

[7]   El-Diasty M, Wareth G, Melzer F, Mustafa S, Sprague LD, Neubauer H. Isolation of *Brucella abortus* and *Brucella melitensis* from Seronegative Cows is a Serious Impediment in Brucellosis Control. Vet Sci 2018; 5(1): 28.
[http://dx.doi.org/10.3390/vetsci5010028] [PMID: 29522464]

[8]   El-Sayed A, Awad W. Brucellosis: Evolution and expected comeback. Int J Vet Sci Med 2018; 6 (Suppl.): S31-5.
[http://dx.doi.org/10.1016/j.ijvsm.2018.01.008] [PMID: 30761318]

[9]   García Casallas JC, Villalobos Monsalve W, Arias Villate SC, Fino Solano IM. Acute liver failure complication of brucellosis infection: a case report and review of the literature. J Med Case Reports 2018; 12(1): 62.
[http://dx.doi.org/10.1186/s13256-018-1576-4] [PMID: 29519244]

CHAPTER 14

Mycetoma: An Infection by the Formation of Grains on Skin

Muhammad Imran Qadir[*] and **Hira Jamil**

Institute of Molecular Biology & Biotechnology, Bahauddin Zakariya University, Multan, Pakistan

Abstract: Mycetoma is a chronic disease characterized by the formation of grains seen in the tropical and sub-tropical areas where the rate of rainfall is less. It is caused by both bacteria and fungi called actinomycetoma and eumycetoma. Swelling on skin, Painless nodules formed in this disease which later formed grains. In advanced stages of the disease, it can lead to amputation. For diagnosis of this disease direct microbiological observation, serological test, and imaging techniques used. For treatment antibiotics and anti-fungal with surgery used depending upon the agent. Herbal drugs can also be used.

Keywords: Antimicrobial, Actinomycetoma, Eumycetoma, Mycetoma.

INTRODUCTION

Mycetoma is a chronic disease characterized by the formation of grains that affect the subcutaneous tissues, bones, and skin. The infection starts from the site of trauma or injury *e.g.* splinter or cut can lead to granulomatous reactions. The spread of this disease starts from the skin facial plane and at later stages can involve bones. It mostly involves foot, but in some cases hand, neck, legs, back, shoulder also involved. It is prevalent in tropical and sub-tropical regions. In Africa, this disease has the highest prevalence. In most cases, this disease occurs in a hot climate and have a short period of rainfall [1]. This disease was first recognized by Gill in 1842 in southern of Madura. Godfrey firstly reported a case of mycetoma in India [2]. Carter classified mycetoma based on causative agents [3]. Mycetoma is mostly found in young adults and males are more affected in this disease than females [4].

[*] **Corresponding author Muhammad Imran Qadir:** Institute of Molecular Biology and Biotechnology, Bahauddin Zakariya University, Multan, Pakistan; Tel: +92-61-9210071; Ext. 1920; Fax: +92-61-9210068; E-mail: mrimranqadir@hotmail.com

Muhammad Imran Qadir (Ed.)
All rights reserved-© 2020 Bentham Science Publishers

Mycetoma is caused by bacteria (actinomycetes) and fungi. It is called as the eumycetoma and actinomycetoma [5]. Actinomycetoma is caused by the aerobic species of the actinomycetes which belongs to genera *Actinomadura,Streptomyces* and *Nocardia* and with the *Actinomadura pelletieri, Actinomadura madurae, Streptomyces somaliensis and Nocardia brasiliensis.* Eumycoticmycetoma is caused by many forms of fungi, from which the most common is *Madurella mycetomatis* [4].

SYMPTOMS

It is a slow-spreading skin infection. In this disease swelling of the skin, pus on the skin, and the small painless nodules formed. With the time these nodules soften and then ulcerates to discharge purulent, viscous fluid containing granules. Eventually, affect the bone and lead to amputation. The granules are different in size, consistency, and color, depending upon the species. Although the color of grain can be indicative of the causative agent, it cannot be the final identification. In past yellow grains were considered indicative of bacterial agents responsible for this disease, so when yellow grains formed treated with the anti-bacterial agents. Now a day, it is reported from some studies that the fungus *Pleurostomophora ochracea* can also produce yellow grain, which represents that it is necessary to identify the causative agent at the species level. The chemical structure of grains is not completely known [4].

DIAGNOSIS

The diagnosis of causative microorganism based on the morphology of grains. It can be done by microscopic observations, serological tests, and imaging technology. Microscopic observation involved evaluation of variation in color, consistency, and size of grain which help in determining causative agent. At present no reliable serological test available, which is reliable however many serological assays have been used such as ELISA, indirect hemagglutination assays, immunoblots, immunodiffusion, and counter immunoelectrophoresis. Ultrasonography and radiology enable the diagnosis of disease extent and involvement of the bone. X rays can also be used [3].

MANAGEMENT

At the initial stage, mycetoma is a curable disease, but when it is at the advanced stage only amputation is only available treatment. Due to the painless progression of the disease, it is diagnosed at the advanced stages. The treatment of mycetoma depends upon the site of infection, etiological agent, and extent of disease. In the case of actinomycetoma usually, antibiotics used while in the case of eumycetoma combination of surgery and anti-fungal used. Most commonly prescribed antibiotics for actinomycetoma are streptomycin plus (either dapsone or TMP-sulfamethoxazole). In the case of eumycetoma, triazole antifungal with the surgical excision of the lesions is done. In severe cases, amputation is the only treatment. The treatment is prolonged and expensive. There is no vaccine available for this disease [5].

Prevention is difficult. Instruct the patients to avoid thorny branches and carrying sticks that have contact with the soil especially in the case when contaminated with the cattle dung.

Researchers and the health care provider believe that wearing shoes can prevent injuries that can cause mycetoma because doing this can protect feet while walk or the work outside in the area where germs that can cause the mycetoma are present in the soil and water. Early diagnosis and the treatment, before the symptom causes a serious effect, can decrease the chances of disabilities due to mycetoma and might cure this condition.

CONSENT FOR PUBLICATION

Not applicable.

CONFLICT OF INTEREST

The authors declare no conflict of interest, financial or otherwise.

ACKNOWLEDGEMENTS

Declared none.

REFERENCES

[1]   Boiron P, Locci R, Goodfellow M, *et al.* Nocardia, nocardiosis and mycetoma. Med Mycol 1998; 36 (Suppl. 1): 26-37.
[PMID: 9988489]

[2]   Isolation of Madurella mycetomi from soil in India. Hindustan antibiotics bulletin 1968; 10(4): 8-314.

[3]   Carter HV. On a new and striking form of fungus disease principally affecting the foot and prevailing endemically in many parts of India. Trans Med Phys Soc Bombay 1860; 6: 104-42.

[4]   Mohamed HT, Fahal A, van de Sande W. Mycetoma: epidemiology, treatment challenges, and progress. Res Rep Trop Med 2015; 6: 31-6.

[5]   McGinnis MR. Mycetoma. Dermatol Clin 1996; 14(1): 97-104.
[http://dx.doi.org/10.1016/S0733-8635(05)70329-6] [PMID: 8821162]

CHAPTER 15

Plague: *Yersinia Pestis* Infection

Muhammad Imran Qadir[*], **Saif Ur Rehman** and **Afshan Saleem**

Institute of Molecular Biology & Biotechnology, Bahauddin Zakariya University, Multan, Pakistan

Abstract: A gram-negative bacterium called *Yersinia pestis* causes plague. Plague is a deadly fatal "disease" and it killed millions of people during its three pandemic outbreaks. Due to the discovery of the causative agent of the plague by Alexandre Yersin, it was named as *Yersinia pestis*. Two types of plagues, bubonic plague, and pneumonic plague are caused by the bacteria. The bacteria use some rodents and fleas as a transmission vector. Fleas need a specific temperature and humidity for its developmental stages. The victim of the plague is not infectious for normal people. Symptoms of bubonic plague include severe headache, bleeding in mouth, restlessness, limb pain, and irritation. Sometimes, Yersinia makes its way to the liver, lungs, spleen, and other organs of the body. The patient feels burning fever and wishes to take a bath with cold water. A rapid diagnostic test is applied to assess the level of disease. An early diagnosis can lead to more chances to cure the disease. Vaccine for the bubonic plague was designed at the start of the last century but it is not efficient rather it is reactogenic. Antibiotics for bubonic plague are more efficient but fail for pneumonic plague.

KeyWords: Antibiotics, Fleas, RDT, Rodents, Vaccine.

INTRODUCTION

Yersinia pestis is the gram-negative bacteria. This strain of bacteria affects the rodents but it also harms the humans causing plague in them. The bacteria are airborne, water-borne, and food-borne. In humans, Bubonic plague and pneumonic plague are caused by the mentioned strain of bacteria. This disease killed 200 million people in the past. The disease is transmitted by fleas in human fellows. When the foregut is blocked by plague bacillus then, it is transmitted to human beings. The bubonic plague spreads mainly through fleas, so, it depends upon the active fleas. Rodents and fleas both are the vectors for the plague involving 200 species and 30 species orderly [1]. The reproduction of fleas depends upon environmental factors because humidity and temperature mainly

---

[*] **Corresponding author Muhammad Imran Qadir:** Institute of Molecular Biology and Biotechnology, Bahauddin Zakariya University, Multan, Pakistan; Tel: 192-61-9210071; Ext. 1920; Fax: 192-61-9210068; E-mail: mrimranqadir@hotmail.com

Muhammad Imran Qadir (Ed.)
All rights reserved-© 2020 Bentham Science Publishers

influence the egg-laying and the progression of larvae. Temperature below 7°C retards the developmental steps and the temperature ranging from 18°C to 27°C and 70% humidity are the best conditions for the development of fleas. Plague disease consists of three major types, pneumonic plague, bubonic plague, and septicemic plague. The pneumonic plague spreads more rapidly and progressively and if not treated early it can lead to the death of its victim. When the patients of pneumonic plague cough, they release airborne droplets which can spread to other people increasing the risk of the disease to the healthy individuals. Plague followed three major pandemics starting from the 6th century and killed millions of people and led to enormous short epidemics and acts as a source to spread other diseases. The very pandemic is thought to be originated in central Asia and then followed other trade pathways. When the disease reached the Mediterranean, it swiftly stormed to Italy, France, and Greece following the sea traffic. Later on, the disease spread to the whole of Europe through the land. The third and major worldwide pandemic occurred when the disease arrived at Canton and Hong Kong. Alexandre Yersin made the first breakthrough in Hong Kong by identifying the plague Bacillus. Due to this attempt, the disease was named *Yersinia pestis* in 1970. Yersin was the very first person who linked plague and rats. He claimed that plague disease has a relation with black rats and the reservoir of black rats was infected before human fellows. However, Hankin and Simond refuted the theory of Yersin by arguing that bacillus can survive only outside the body of victims and it is rarely recoverable from the victims. Ogata and Simond working independently discovered the role of fleas as the transmission vector of the plague [2] Fig. (**6**).

SYMPTOMS

Infected flea-bitten patients suffering from bubonic plague are not serious infectious to the normal persons, so they could be placed and nursed in the general ward. The start of symptoms appears after two to six days when the temperature of the victim rises to 38.8°C–39.4°C and the patient feels rigors, chills, and severe type of headache and the splitting pain in the abdomen, limbs, and back. The symptoms also include an acute type of lymphadenitis that occur in lymph nodes and then spreading to the liver, spleen, and the other organs of the body. Plague is present in the world even today though reasons are not there to explain it [3]. The patients feel restlessness, confusion, irritation and mostly vomit. Death occurs in most cases in three to six days. They may recover if they are lucky enough to survive on the seventh day. In 5% of victims of bubonic plague, Yersinia makes its way to lungs and the sputum of the victim contains bacteria when he coughs out, leading to the transfer of bacteria to a healthy person who is very close to the patient and making him also a prey. The patients cannot walk and move to some distance. Without any treatment, they die in three to six days. During the Athens plague, the victims felt a severe kind of headaches, bulging eyes, and bleeding that occurred from the throats and mouths. They also suffered heavy coughing and chest pains. Unquenchable thirst, diarrhea, vomiting, and stomach cramping also appeared. The blisters and small brakes occupied the skin. The victim preferred to dive in cold and chilled water due to burning in high-temperature fever and he wished to go naked [4 - 7].

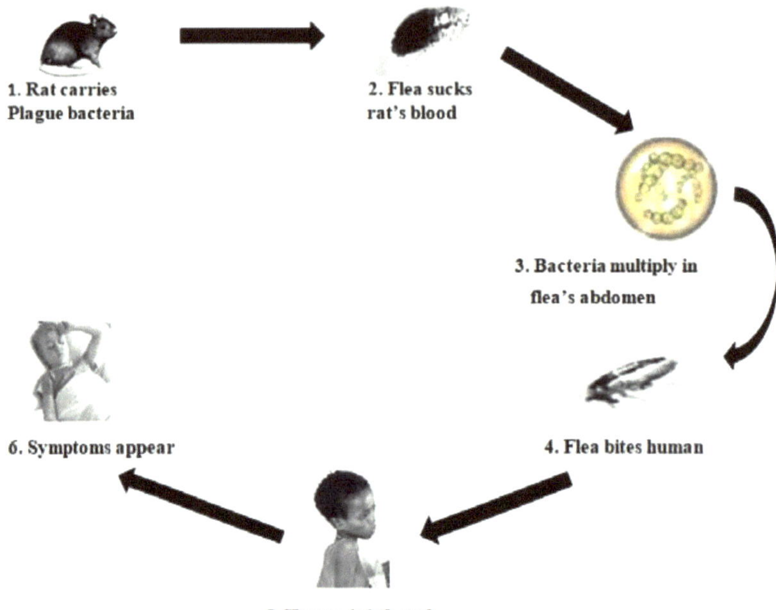

Fig. (6). Transmission of plague.

DIAGNOSTIC TEST

Plague is a deadly fatal disease if not treated appropriately. Poor people and the remote populations are their prey. Human death and the outbreak of disease is also facilitated by late diagnosis. A rapid diagnostic test is also applied to assess the disease level. Rapid diagnosis test uses the monoclonal antibodies that were produced against F1 antigens of *Yersinia pestis*. From the available samples, specificity and sensitivity were judged and these were compared with the calculations from tests for the disease and the findings of ELISA.

Rapid diagnosis test is much reliable, target-specific, more sensitive, very rapid for the diagnosis of bubonic and pneumonic plague, and can be performed easily by some workers. The test would be more helpful in endemic countries to limit the plague [8].

VACCINE

A vaccine against *Yersinia pestis* is available in the world from the start of the previous century. This vaccine consists of killed whole-cell and lives attenuated particles but it also has many problems. The vaccine which is live attenuated is very risky and reactogenic. Moreover, the vaccine has not been licensed to apply to humans. Such type of vaccine gives poor protection for the pneumonic plague and boosting up the immune system requires repeated and multiple doses. Using the live attenuated vaccine mechanism, many other candidate vaccines have been prepared, *e.g.* naked DNA vaccine, subunit vaccine, and rationally attenuated mutants, *etc.* Out of the mentioned types of vaccines, the subunit vaccine provides a better result to be proved as a vaccine because it protects against pneumonic plague as well as bubonic plague [8].

ANTIBIOTICS

Antibiotic treatment for Bubonic plague is usually effective but as far as the pneumonic plague is concerned, it is very difficult to treat it through antibiotics and it leads to death in most of the cases. The clinical signs of plague in rats resembled those in humans as in the case of Bubonic plague.

CONSENT FOR PUBLICATION

Not applicable.

CONFLICT OF INTEREST

The authors declare no conflict of interest, financial or otherwise.

ACKNOWLEDGEMENTS

Declared none.

REFERENCES

[1]   Duncan CJ, Scott S. What caused the black death? Postgrad Med J 2005; 81(955): 315-20.
        [http://dx.doi.org/10.1136/pgmj.2004.024075] [PMID: 15879045]

[2]   Hinnebusch BJ. Bubonic plague: a molecular genetic case history of the emergence of an infectious disease. J Mol Med (Berl) 1997; 75(9): 645-52.
        [http://dx.doi.org/10.1007/s001090050148] [PMID: 9351703]

[3]   Hinnebusch BJ, Perry RD, Schwan TG. Role of the *Yersinia pestis* hemin storage (hms) locus in the transmission of plague by fleas. Science 1996; 273(5273): 367-70.
        [http://dx.doi.org/10.1126/science.273.5273.367] [PMID: 8662526]

[4]   Popov S. Plague (*Yersinia pestis*). Encyclopedia of Bioterrorism Defense 2011.

[5]   Titball R, Hill J, Lawton D, Brown K. *Yersinia pestis* and plague. Portland Press Limited. 2003.
        [http://dx.doi.org/10.1042/bst0310104]

[6]   Titball RW, Williamson ED. *Yersinia pestis* (plague) vaccines. Expert Opin Biol Ther 2004; 4(6): 965-73.
[http://dx.doi.org/10.1517/14712598.4.6.965] [PMID: 15174978]

[7]   Zietz BP, Dunkelberg H. The history of the plague and the research on the causative agent *Yersinia pestis*. Int J Hyg Environ Health 2004; 207(2): 165-78.
[http://dx.doi.org/10.1078/1438-4639-00259] [PMID: 15031959]

[8]   Sebbane F, Gardner D, Long D, Gowen BB, Hinnebusch BJ. Kinetics of disease progression and host response in a rat model of bubonic plague. Am J Pathol 2005; 166(5): 1427-39.
[http://dx.doi.org/10.1016/S0002-9440(10)62360-7] [PMID: 15855643]

CHAPTER 16

MRSA Infections: Methicillin-Resistant *Staphylococcus Aureus* Infections

Muhammad Imran Qadir[*] and **Shahpara Rehman**

Institute of Molecular Biology & Biotechnology, Bahauddin Zakariya University, Multan, Pakistan

Abstract: Methicillin resistant *Staphylococcus aureus* (MRSA) stays as one of the most vituperative human pathogens and has been documented recently in veterinary settings also. The prevalent use of antibiotics both in human and veterinary medication resulted in the appearance of resistant strains of *S. aureus*. Resistance to methicillin is resolute by *mecA* gene, encoding affinity less penicillin-binding protein PBP 2. Cohort animals, counting dogs, cats, horses, small foreign animals, wildlife animals, and farm animals may comprise a pool for MRSA transmission to humans and others. The appearance, risk factors for MRSA transmission among colonized or infected animals, and possible treatment for infection control are reviewed in the present paper.

Keywords: Close Contacts, Escort Animals, Inspection, Morbidity, MRSA, Prevalence, Transience.

INTRODUCTION

Methicillin-resistant *Staphylococcus aureus* (MRSA) are types of *Staphylococcus* bacteria that are unaffected by beta-lactam antibiotics, including penicillin, ampicillin, amoxicillin, methicillin, cephalosporin & monobactams. Staph bacteria live on the skin and in the nose generally exclusive of causing problems. It cannot be treated with common antibiotics such as methicillin so it is different from other types of bacteria. They are problematic only when grounds infection in any species. These infections turn into serious in a week and ill people. This pathogen is mostly present among humans and animals. Staph's strains known as MRSA are arduous to treat as they do not retort to common antibiotics used to eradicate bacteria. It becomes hardest to remove the infection when strong antibiotics such as methicillin do not influence bacteria. Using antibiotics repeatedly and not in the right way is the leading cause of MRSA emergence. As

[*] **Corresponding author Muhammad Imran Qadir:** Institute of Molecular Biology and Biotechnology, Bahauddin Zakariya University, Multan, Pakistan; Tel: +92-61-9210071; Ext. 1920; Fax: +92-61-9210068; E-mail: mrimranqadir@hotmail.com

Muhammad Imran Qadir (Ed.)
All rights reserved-© 2020 Bentham Science Publishers

time passes antibiotics no longer work well on bacteria as bacteria become resistant to them, So MRSA is termed as "superbugs". Ogston and Rosenbach discovered it the first time in 1882, from that time it stays as a very affluent bacterium. From the mid-1940s it shows a continuous advancement in terms of antibiotic resistance, as beta-lactam producing strains were resolute. *S. aureus* is found on the genomic islands of the chromosome, which are mobile genetic elements and are classified according to the place of their attachment site and the progression process of their integrase gene. MRSA impose serious trouble not only in medical & economic cost but also cause numerous morbidity & transience. In Europe MRSA infections roughly affect more than 150,000 patients annually causing the extra cost of 380 million in healthcare units [1].

HISTORICAL BACKGROUND OF MRSA

MRSA was first reported in 1960 and in these days are acting as a chief hospital-acquired pathogen globally. A brief timeline for the emergence of MRSA has been described in Table **1**.

Table 1. Timeline for the emergence of MRSA.

1929	Fleming reported fungal contaminant producing penicillin
World war I & II	Penicillin remained as a major drug against *S. aureus.*
1940	Beta-lactam enzyme discovered in *E. coli* naming penicillinase
1944	Penicillinase production in *S. aureus*
1948	50% of hospital patient found to be resistant to penicillin
1959	Methicillin introduction which was resistant to penicillinase-resistant penicillin
1960	Methicillin resistant strain was introduced
1962	The epidemic occurred in hospitals
1968	United States recorded the first outbreak of MRSA
1970	*S. aureus* strains become resistant to most penicillinase
1972	MRSA isolated in mastitic cow
2004-12	MRSA isolated in domestic and wild animals

CAUSES

MRSA stretches through casual contact or unhygienic objects like all other staph bacteria transmission. It normally extends from the hands of MRSA suffering that might be anyone from health care setting or society. Unlike the flu virus, MRSA does not spread through the air until a person has pneumonia and coughing. Hospital gained MRSA is called healthcare-associated methicillin resistant

Staphylococcus aureus. Healthcare-associated methicillin resistant *Staphylococcus aureus* occurs mostly in sick persons with a destabilized immune system and infection mostly happens in wounds, burns, eyes, blood, or other sites where tubes enter the body. In the past, MRSA tainted only ill people but now MRSA is widespread more in healthy people who have lesion or abrasion and those who are in physical contact.

On the skin and in the nose of hale and hearty people *Staphylococcus aureus* is mostly found. Strains of *Staphylococcus aureus* possess ß lactamase substance making them resistant that degrades penicillin by killing its antibacterial activity. Antibiotic methicillin is a type of penicillin that was developed in the early 1960s [2].

LABORATORY DIAGNOSIS

MRSA detection and categorization have been done based on new swift techniques. In laboratories for the detection of MRSA strains, real-time PCR and quantitative PCR is using mostly. Solid agar media for screening cannot be used commonly. Multiplexed PCR primer is a molecular method that detects precise genes for *S. aureus*. Phenotypic methods for *S. aureus* recognition are Gram staining and coagulase tests. Genes of *S. aureus* can be finding out by Oxacillin & cefoxitin test. Pulsed-field gel electrophoresis is a molecular typing method used in detection [2].

ANTIBIOTICS ACTIVITY AGAINST MRSA

Antibiotics using for the treatment of MRSA is one topical agent, a restricted number of oral agents and numerous agents for intravenous (IV) infusion.

Topical Agents

Mupirocin is used as a topical agent to treat *S. aureus* infections and it works by inhibiting bacterial protein and ribonucleic acid production.

Oral Agents

Oral therapies frequently used in the treatment are tetracycline, linezolid, clindamycin, and rifampin and they work by inhibiting bacterial protein production.

Oral and Intravenous Agents

In oral and IV form Linezolid & Clindamycin are accessible. Due to certain advantages, such as it is availability to body easily after oral organization, pierce into skin and skin structures, active in high bacterial infection clindamycin is used as primary treatment for community-acquired MRSA. Manufacture of virulence factors in MRSA is also inhibited by using it. Clindamycin acts on bacterial ribosome so unable it to work by inhibiting protein synthesis. But unfortunately, sometimes due to methylase production that changes the ribosomal sites to produce protein MRSA develops resistance to clindamycin.

Intravenous Agents

For many years vancomycin is used as a major treatment of MRSA. Vancomycin is a glycopeptide and it performs its function by preventing cell wall synthesis. Vancomycin is using habitually as MRSA strains develop resistance mechanisms against antibiotics. Teicoplanin is a structurally analogue to vancomycin, used as a substitute for the treatment of Gram-positive infections, such as MRSA. Due to longer half-life and less serum level, teicoplanin over vancomycin is beneficial.

Treatment of Skin and Soft Tissue Infections

Due to high resistance rate, Fluoroquinolones *e.g.* Ciprofloxacin, and macrolides *e.g.* erythromycin, azithromycin, clarithromycin, are not recommended as the treatment of MRSA. Due to antimicrobial resistance, toxicity, great potential for inappropriate use, and cost linezolid are not mostly used. The accumulation of rifampin or another inclined antibiotic should be sturdily calculated when quinolones are permitted for MRSA infections [3].

CONTROL CHALLENGES

Antibiotic resistance in humans and animals can be controlled by the conniving of opposing strains through vulnerability tests and decolonization of carriers. Effective antibiotics in the treatment of CA MRSA infection are clindamycin, doxycycline, and trimethoprim sulphameth. For concealed use in the treatment of MRSA infection fosfomycin and fusidic acid are under investigation. *Streptococcus pneumonia* and *Hemophilus influenza* are used in the first attempt to develop the first vaccine for *S. aureus*. The formula used for it called Staphax developed by biopharmaceuticals in the 1990s although it remains unsuccessful.

Infection Control - Primary Avoidance

Primary prevention is the execution of screening, infection control, treatment, and managerial actions intended to decrease and identify the frequency of MRSA infections in the population. Staff should be provided information on the transmission, anticipation, treatment, and suppression of MRSA infections. MRSA conduction can be prevented by regular hand washing. Antimicrobial soaps with triclosan are suitable to reduce skin flora as plain liquid soap is effective. Personal defending tools must be used *e.g.* gloves to shield hands & gowns to evade sprays and splashes among people who are in close contact with each other. On exposed surfaces, diluted bleach solution or EPA registered disinfectant should be used. To reduce the development of antibiotic resistance the gratuitous use of broad-spectrum antibiotics should be truncated [4].

Infection Control - Secondary Prevention

Infection control, amplified screening, cure and directorial procedures intended to control MRSA infections are the execution of secondary prevention. All procedures that were adopted in primary prevention should be sustained all through secondary prevention. Education should be given to patients concerning infection. Educational information can be given in the written form using proper lingo, and the information should be cautiously described.

CONCLUSION

Chemotherapy and control measures are being disturbed by the extensive circulation of numerous drug-resistant strains and bacterial clones. MRSA infection is not only spreading through hospitals but also in communities during contact with tame and untamed animals as well as foodstuffs and the surroundings. Ample policy framework is needed on infection control of MRSA as well as strict accomplishment of such a control program to check the extent of MRSA infections. To check auxiliary confrontation by microorganisms, efficient control of MRSA, and the impediment of haphazard use of antibiotics is desired Selective screening & isolation programs can be effectively used to control the dominance of MRSA.

CONSENT FOR PUBLICATION

Not applicable.

CONFLICT OF INTEREST

The authors declare no conflict of interest, financial or otherwise.

ACKNOWLEDGEMENTS

Declared none.

REFERENCES

[1]   Akande AO. Global trend of Methicillin-resistant *staphylococcus aureus* and emerging challenges for control: a review. Afr J Clin Exp Microbiol 2010; 11(3): 150-8.

[2]   Batabyal B, Kundu G, Biswas S. Methicillin resistant *Staphylococcus aureus* (MRSA): a review. Int Res J Biol Sci 2012; 1(7): 65-71.

[3]   Grema HA, Geidam YA, Gadzama GB, Ameh JA, Suleiman A. Methicillin resistant *Staphylococcus aureus* (MRSA): a review. Adv Anim Vet Sci 2015; 3(2): 79-98.
        [http://dx.doi.org/10.14737/journal.aavs/2015/3.2.79.98]

[4]   Baillargeon J, Kelley MF, Leach CT, Baillargeon G, Pollock BH. Methicillin-resistant *Staphylococcus aureus* infection in the Texas prison system. Clin Infect Dis 2004; 38(9): e92-5.
        [http://dx.doi.org/10.1086/383146] [PMID: 15127360]

CHAPTER 17

Otitis Media: An Inflammation of the Ear

Muhammad Imran Qadir[*] and **Fahad Zafar**

Institute of Molecular Biology & Biotechnology, Bahauddin Zakariya University, Multan, Pakistan

Abstract: Otitis media is the most occurring disease in Childs regarding bacterial infections especially *streptococcus* pneumonia. Monitoring of these disease-causing agents is necessary to generate new means of treatment, vaccines, and precautionary measures. This chapter will show different methods of diagnosis either based on symptoms or with the help of other means, also the treatment policy by using antibiotics or other options such as surgery are discussed along with the precautionary measures that are to be taken to prevent the Children from such a serious disease.

Keywords: Management, Otitis Media, *streptococcus* pneumonia.

INTRODUCTION

Otitis can be defined as the inflammation of the ear. Mostly middle part of the ear is affected so it can be named Otitis Media. Otitis Media is characterized by severe pain and swelling on the ear usually in children [1 - 4].

CAUSES

The origin of this disease mostly correlates with the Bacterial infection in the throat that can be extended to the ear and cause inflammation of the ear. It can also be of viral infection (influenza, rhinovirus, adenovirus, and coronavirus). Mostly bacteria *streptococcus pneumoniae, Moraxella cattarhalis*, non-typeable *Haemophilus influenzae,* and Group A *streptococcus* are involved in this infection [5, 6].

[*] **Corresponding author Muhammad Imran Qadir:** Institute of Molecular Biology and Biotechnology, Bahauddin Zakariya University, Multan, Pakistan; Tel: +92-61-9210071; Ext. 1920; Fax: +92-61-9210068; E-mail: mrimranqadir@hotmail.com

Muhammad Imran Qadir (Ed.)
All rights reserved-© 2020 Bentham Science Publishers

SYMPTOMS

The following symptoms can be observed in the case of Otitis Media [7, 8].

- Severe pain in the ear and the surrounding region
- Swelling
- Fever
- Temporary hearing loss
- Permanent hearing loss may occur if it is not treated
- Disability in speaking and language problem may occur due to hearing loss
- Consistent drainage of fluid from the ear
- Lack of balance *etc.*

DIAGNOSIS

The following tools can be used for the diagnosis of Otitis Media in children [9].

A common or frequent way to diagnose the Otitis Media (infection) is to observe the ear of the patient with an otoscope that assists the physician to observe the eardrum and outer ear with light provided by the otoscope. Inflammation (redness, swelling, hot, pain) will indicate the infection.

A pneumatic otoscope can also be used for its diagnosis by blowing a puff of air on the eardrum to check the movement of the eardrum. If liquid or fluid is present behind the eardrum due to infection, the eardrum will not show such a movement that is present when there is a presence of air behind the eardrum. So with the help of the pneumatic otoscope physician can diagnose Otitis Media.

Tympanometry is also a test to diagnose the Otitis media by observing inflammation (showing infection) of the middle ear by inserting a small, very soft plug containing device to change the air pressure in the ear canal. Also, a speaker and microphone are the parts of tympanometry

MANAGEMENT

In management practices, the following tools may be used to tackle that problem or disease [10, 11].

- Treatment Otitis media can be efficiently treated by using antibiotics until recovery. If there is a problem of bacterial resistance against the available antibiotics then the option of treatment with several antibiotics should have to be used so that these medicines can act synergistically to overcome the problem of resistance presented by the bacteria. Another problem can occur in the form of side effects of such drugs or medicines that are going to be used such as vomiting like conditions and diarrhea *etc.*

- Myringotomy Hearing loss may occur if fluid sustains for more than three months behind the eardrum due to infection so, an operation named as myringotomy is done to remove that fluid including the insertion of small but very soft tubes of plastic in the opening of eardrum to maintain pressure between inside the ear and outer environment after giving the anesthetic drug. Metal tubes can also be used depending upon the conditions and recommendations of the physician. These tubes can be removed after 6-12 months. Hearing should be restored properly after the removal of fluid. The operation can be repeated in such a case when there is a return of otitis media including the fluid production behind the eardrum. After the operation, it should be informed to prevent the entry of water in the ear while bathing and swimming by applying a plug.
- Prevention Availability of certain vaccines can assist to control such type of cases.

CONSENT FOR PUBLICATION

Not applicable.

CONFLICT OF INTEREST

The authors declare no conflict of interest, financial or otherwise.

ACKNOWLEDGEMENTS

Declared none.

REFERENCES

[1]   Berman S, Byrns PJ, Bondy J, Smith PJ, Lezotte D. Otitis media-related antibiotic prescribing patterns, outcomes, and expenditures in a pediatric medicaid population. Pediatrics 1997; 100(4): 585-92.
[http://dx.doi.org/10.1542/peds.100.4.585] [PMID: 9310510]

[2]   Culpepper L, Froom J. Routine antimicrobial treatment of acute otitis media: is it necessary? JAMA 1997; 278(20): 1643-5.

[3]   Dagan R, Leibovitz E, Leiberman A, Yagupsky P. Clinical significance of antibiotic resistance in acute otitis media and implication of antibiotic treatment on carriage and spread of resistant organisms. Pediatr Infect Dis J 2000; 19(5) (Suppl.): S57-65.
[http://dx.doi.org/10.1097/00006454-200005001-00009] [PMID: 10821473]

[4]   Dowell SF, Butler JC, Giebink GS, *et al.* Acute otitis media: management and surveillance in an era of pneumococcal resistance--a report from the Drug-resistant *streptococcus pneumoniae* Therapeutic Working Group. Pediatr Infect Dis J 1999; 18(1): 1-9.
[http://dx.doi.org/10.1097/00006454-199901000-00002] [PMID: 9951971]

[5]   Glasziou PP, Hayem M, Del Mar CB. Antibiotics for acute otitis media in children. Cochrane Database Syst Rev 2000; 2: CD000219.
[http://dx.doi.org/10.1002/14651858.CD000219]

[6]   Kozyrskyj AL, Hildes-Ripstein GE, Longstaffe SE, *et al.* Treatment of acute otitis media with a shortened course of antibiotics: a meta-analysis. JAMA 1998; 279(21): 1736-42.
[http://dx.doi.org/10.1001/jama.279.21.1736] [PMID: 9624028]

[7]   Maw R, Wilks J, Harvey I, Peters TJ, Golding J. Early surgery compared with watchful waiting for glue ear and effect on language development in preschool children: a randomised trial. Lancet 1999; 353(9157): 960-3.
[http://dx.doi.org/10.1016/S0140-6736(98)05295-7] [PMID: 10459904]

[8]   Otitis Media with Effusion in Young Children, Clinical Practice Guideline No. 12, AHCPR Publication No. 94-0622. Agency for Healthcare Research and Quality, Rockville, MD July.

[9]   Pichichero ME. Acute otitis media: part II. Treatment in an era of increasing antibiotic resistance. Am Fam Physician 2000; 61(8): 2410-6.
[PMID: 10794582]

[10]   Rosenfeld RM, Vertrees JE, Carr J, *et al.* Clinical efficacy of antimicrobial drugs for acute otitis media: a meta-analysis of 5400 children from thirty-three randomized trials 1994.
[http://dx.doi.org/10.1016/S0022-3476(94)70356-6]

[11]   Stine AR. Is amoxicillin more effective than placebo in treating acute otitis media in children younger than 2 years? J Fam Pract 2000; 49(5): 465-6.
[PMID: 10836781]

CHAPTER 18

Yaws Disease: A *Treponema Pallidum* Infection

Muhammad Imran Qadir[*] and **Rahat Bano**

Institute of Molecular Biology & Biotechnology, Bahauddin Zakariya University, Multan, Pakistan

Abstract: Yaws disease is an infectious disease which is caused by *Treponema pallidum*. It is an endemic non-venereal disease. In the tropical regions where humidity is present yaws are spread by skin to skin contact. The main camping was started to eradicate this disease by using injectable penicillin. It mainly affects children who are living in poor areas they resultantly suffered from lesions of the bone, cartilage, and skin. The reinfection risk caused by repetitive contact with those children who have an infection and they seem to be a key factor in predicting the treatment failure.

Keywords: Intramuscular Injection, Penicillin G Benzathine, *Treponema pallidum*, Yaws Disease.

INTRODUCTION

Yaw is an infectious disease it is a debilitating disease that mainly affects the children especially in the rural areas and in the tropical regions [1]. Yaws can easily be treated with antibiotics and present in the World Health Organization's eradication list. Yaws is a disease which is caused by the bacteria called Yaws, *Treponema pallidum* [2].

CAUSE

It is one of the endemic non-venereal diseases caused by *Treponema pallidum* [3]. Earlier, yaws were common all over the tropics [4] In the tropical regions where humidity is present Yaws is spread by skin-to-skin contact. The clinical indexes for syphilis show that syphilis does not transmit from mother-to-child [5]. *T. pallidum* is the main pathogen, studied in humans that have evaded in the *Vitro* cultivation [6].

[*] **Corresponding author Muhammad Imran Qadir:** Institute of Molecular Biology and Biotechnology, Bahauddin Zakariya University, Multan, Pakistan; Tel: +92-61-9210071; Ext. 1920; Fax: +92-61-9210068; E-mail: mrimranqadir@hotmail.com

Muhammad Imran Qadir (Ed.)
All rights reserved-© 2020 Bentham Science Publishers

PREVALENCE

In the 1950s and 1960s, the main camping was started to eradicate the yaws, by using injectable penicillin, yaws were treated and reduced the number of cases by 95% worldwide, but in recent years, yaws has again reappeared in Africa, Asia, and the western Pacific. In 2012, it has been seen that in the treatment of the disease one oral dose of azithromycin was effective as compared to the intramuscular penicillin, and WHO launched a new initiative to eliminate yaws by 2020 [5].

SYMPTOMS

It mainly affects children who are living in poor areas they resultantly suffered from lesions of the bone, cartilage, and skin. The untreated disease can cause destructive lessons in the bones and cartilage [4]. In bones, Yaws disease was studied for clinical and X-rays aspects. Some patients were suffering from yaws disease having multiple symmetries or no-symmetry papules and nodes on their skin. They have a systematic toxic symptom. Patients who have Yaws disease, they have brown abscess under the extremities of the skin. Surrounding the ulcer they also have multiple bayberry-like nodes up and down surrounding the ulcer. The bone lesions were predominantly periosteal proliferation and hyperostosis. The lesions on the bone were hyperostosis and destroy the bone. With the help of the CDC, lesion samples were tested by using multiple numbers of the real-time PCR assay. In the start, samples were tested for the identification of bacteria *T. pallidum* DNA [7]. If the result of PCR was positive for *T. pallidum* subsp. *pertenue* then the second multiplex RT PCR procedure is performed to check that 23S rRNA becomes mutated or not, because of this gene related to the resistance of azithromycin. These samples were also tested with the help of a duplex RT PCR for the recognition of *Haemophilus ducreyi* and *Mycobacterium ulcerans* [8]. All the test of the laboratory was performed for the clinical findings. 6 months to 15 years children were conformed serologically to diagnosis the yaws disease, by using the computer-generated randomization sequence. This result described the cure rate and show that 6 months treatment decrease in rapid plasma re-agitate and within 2 weeks applicant who has primary ulcers, also by epithelialization of lesions [9].

MANAGEMENT

It is thought that it is very difficult to resolve chronic infection [10]. Even though it has been reported that penicillin treatment is failed for yaws disease [11] until the resistance for penicillin has not been proven. Maximum medical well-defined treatment becomes failing due to two reasons first reinfection after treatment and second are patient-to-patient variations.

A series of experiments perform which was based on mass-treatment which is done with intramuscular penicillin. In 1996-97, in India Yaws Eradication Program was launched. At the start, the YEP was used as a pilot study in Koraput district, and then later on extensively study in ten states and cover the 49 districts. The goal of the study is to eliminate the disease from the country [12]. It is trying to eradicate the Yaws but it has not yet been eliminated from many terrestrial areas, though, it is already rising in some countries. The disease is not a household disease but somewhat, the transmission of the yaws in the children is a community, public place, or the school. More programs will be needed for the elimination of the yaws disease and need of information to deliver and administer drugs in secluded and under-resourced communities [13].

CONSENT FOR PUBLICATION

Not applicable.

CONFLICT OF INTEREST

The authors declare no conflict of interest, financial or otherwise.

ACKNOWLEDGEMENTS

Declared none.

REFERENCES

[1]   Boock AU, Awah PK, Mou F, Nichter M. Yaws resurgence in Bankim, Cameroon: The relative effectiveness of different means of detection in rural communities. PLoS Negl Trop Dis 2017; 11(5)e0005557
[http://dx.doi.org/10.1371/journal.pntd.0005557] [PMID: 28481900]

[2]   Mitjà O, Houinei W, Moses P, *et al.* Mass treatment with single-dose azithromycin for yaws. N Engl J Med 2015; 372(8): 703-10.
[http://dx.doi.org/10.1056/NEJMoa1408586] [PMID: 25693010]

[3]   Ghinai R, El-Duah P, Chi K-H, *et al.* A cross-sectional study of 'yaws' in districts of Ghana which have previously undertaken azithromycin mass drug administration for trachoma control. PLoS Negl Trop Dis 2015; 9(1)e0003496
[http://dx.doi.org/10.1371/journal.pntd.0003496] [PMID: 25632942]

[4]   Kazadi WM, Asiedu KB, Agana N, Mitjà O. Epidemiology of yaws: an update. Clin Epidemiol 2014; 6: 119-28.
[PMID: 24729728]

[5]   Mitjà O, Hays R, Ipai A, *et al.* Single-dose azithromycin *versus* benzathine benzylpenicillin for treatment of yaws in children in Papua New Guinea: an open-label, non-inferiority, randomised trial. Lancet 2012; 379(9813): 342-7.
[http://dx.doi.org/10.1016/S0140-6736(11)61624-3] [PMID: 22240407]

[6]   Stamm LV. Global challenge of antibiotic-resistant *Treponema pallidum.* Antimicrob Agents Chemother 2010; 54(2): 583-9.
[http://dx.doi.org/10.1128/AAC.01095-09] [PMID: 19805553]

[7]   Chi K-H, Danavall D, Taleo F, *et al.* Molecular differentiation of *Treponema pallidum* subspecies in skin ulceration clinically suspected as yaws in Vanuatu using real-time multiplex PCR and serological methods. Am J Trop Med Hyg 2015; 92(1): 134-8.
[http://dx.doi.org/10.4269/ajtmh.14-0459] [PMID: 25404075]

[8]   Marks M, Chi K-H, Vahi V, *et al. Haemophilus ducreyi* associated with skin ulcers among children, Solomon Islands. Emerg Infect Dis 2014; 20(10): 1705-7.
[http://dx.doi.org/10.3201/eid2010.140573] [PMID: 25271477]

[9]   Parkes R, Renton A, Meheus A, Laukamm-Josten U. Review of current evidence and comparison of guidelines for effective syphilis treatment in Europe. Int J STD AIDS 2004; 15(2): 73-88.
[http://dx.doi.org/10.1258/095646204322764253] [PMID: 15006068]

[10]   Landersdorfer CB, Bulitta JB, Kinzig M, Holzgrabe U, Sörgel F. Penetration of antibacterials into bone: pharmacokinetic, pharmacodynamic and bioanalytical considerations. Clin Pharmacokinet 2009; 48(2): 89-124.
[http://dx.doi.org/10.2165/00003088-200948020-00002] [PMID: 19271782]

[11]   Backhouse JL, Hudson BJ, Hamilton PA, Nesteroff SI. Failure of penicillin treatment of yaws on Karkar Island, Papua New Guinea. Am J Trop Med Hyg 1998; 59(3): 388-92.
[http://dx.doi.org/10.4269/ajtmh.1998.59.388] [PMID: 9749630]

[12]   Bora D, Dhariwal AC, Lal S. Yaws and its eradication in India--a brief review. J Commun Dis 2005; 37(1): 1-11.
[PMID: 16637394]

[13]   Mitjà O, Hays R, Ipai A, *et al.* Outcome predictors in treatment of yaws. Emerg Infect Dis 2011; 17(6): 1083-5.
[http://dx.doi.org/10.3201/eid/1706.101575] [PMID: 21749808]

CHAPTER 19

Pharyngitis: An Inflammation of the Throat

Muhammad Imran Qadir[*] and **Jaleel Ahmad**

Institute of Molecular Biology & Biotechnology, Bahauddin Zakariya University, Multan, Pakistan

Abstract: Pharyngitis is a throat infection and the back throat inflammation causes throat infection and it is a common reason to visit physicians. Swallowing may be uncomfortable and painful. Commonly, throat infection symptoms are illness, like the flu or cold. In this review, we have discussed the national perspective, epidemiology, regional perspective, clinical diagnosis, pathogenesis, clinical presentation, and causes of inflammation pharynges.

Keywords: A Respiratory Infection, Pharyngitis, Sore Throat.

INTRODUCTION

In most cases, the viral origin of throat infection however microbial etiology is described and in the Group A *streptococcus* bacteria cause of severe pharyngitis [1]. Severe throat infection is an inflammation disorder considered by swelling, heat, redness, and pain. Word Throat infection frequently used to define laryngitis, tonsillitis, and pharyngitis that happen for a short period, which affects respiratory tract infection. Mainly four regions larynx, pharynx epiglottis, and tonsils are involved. Anyhow normal of an epidemic influenza time, a mature may be infected with influenza two to three times in one year [2]. Throat infection by non-infective normally caused by the change of environment like air pollution, low humidity, smoking, and change in temperature. Throat infection has an important effect on the usual regular functioning and activities of a patient, including eating, talking, swallowing, concentration, and sleeping. The literature of throat infection indicates that infection of bacteria does not cause of throat infection caused by group A bacteria B-hemolytic *streptococcus* (*streptococcus pyogenes*) contribution to almost 20% of all total throat infection and throat infection in mature. Approximately 80% of a throat infection in mature is

[*] **Corresponding author Muhammad Imran Qadir:** Institute of Molecular Biology and Biotechnology, Bahauddin Zakariya University, Multan, Pakistan; Tel: +92-61-9210071; Ext. 1920; Fax: +92-61-9210068; E-mail: mrimranqadir@hotmail.com

Muhammad Imran Qadir (Ed.)
All rights reserved-© 2020 Bentham Science Publishers

produced by influenza virus critical respiratory syndrome respirational syncytial virus, rhinovirus, and coronavirus. Therefore, antibiotics are commonly not the first treatment for severe throat infection. Treatment of throat infection by prescribed antibiotics and guideline of the World Health Organization have discouraged prescription antibiotics [3]. Moreover, the prescription of antibiotic decreases would decrease the produce resistance of antibiotics in the public and decrease the total charge problem on the healthcare system.

SYMPTOMS

Many ways of throat infection affect an individual and symptoms of throat infection differ from person to person. Therefore, particular define disorder symptoms as a feel tickling and scorching feeling in the throat. Throat infection affects the person as a common pain sensation that starts at the oral back and slowly increases in the area of the central throat Fig. (7). In many circumstances of severe throat infection no signs of problems, like difficulty in breathing and prolonged fever conventionally without antibiotics may be managed [4, 5].

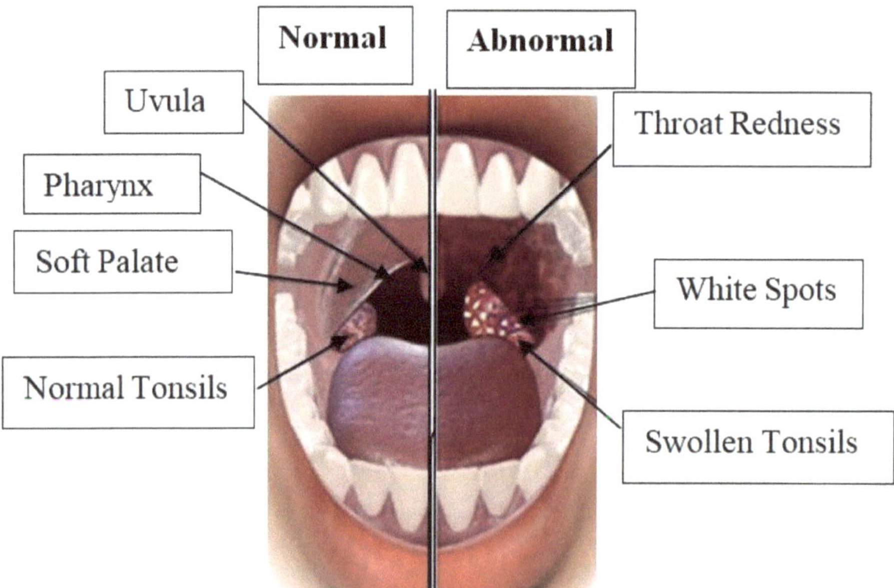

Fig. (7). Throat infection.

DIAGNOSIS

Culture of *Streptococci* through the swab throat from an upper respiratory tract to diagnose the pharyngitis of severe *streptococcal*. The sensitivity of single swab throat culture has 90 to 95% to detect the group A hemolytic *streptococci* in the upper respiratory tract and numerous variables affect the results of throat culture accuracy. The technique in which the Impact of a secured swab important on *streptococci* yields from culture.

Swab throat samples would be taken from both tonsillar or tonsilsupper pharyngeal wall and fossae. Mouth and oral pharynx areas are not suitable sites, and swab would not be touch these sites already or after the suitable parts have been tested. If a patient takes antibiotics already or at the time of swab throat gained and obtained results should be negative-false.

It has been stated that the use of selective culture media and anaerobic incubation can enhance the results of positive culture proportion. Though, data are incompatible concerning the effect of the environment of culture media and incubation, in the lack of a certain advantage, the effort and increased cost related with selective culture media and usage of anaerobe incubation are problematic to validate, especially for physicians who procedure throat culture [6]. The clinical importance of many of the colonies of group A β-hemolytic *streptococcal* present on the culture plate of the throat is difficult. However, patients with an exact severe group A *streptococcal* pharyngitis are expected to have positive and strong cultures as compare to *streptococcus* carrier patients. The results of throat culture too much overlap distinction cannot be made alone on this basis exactly.

MANAGEMENT

These reflect historical and not current immunological actions and are not significant in the severe pharyngitis diagnosis. They are significant for confirmation of earlier infections of *streptococcal* in patients assumed to have post-*streptococcal* severe glomerulonephritis or severe rheumatic fever. They are also useful in likely studies of epidemiological, for differentiating patients with severe infection from carrier patients. The foremost purpose uses antibiotics for the treatment of pharyngitis and throat infection to avoid rheumatic fever. Meanwhile, in the population occurrence of rheumatic fever is low, and has less over the last 30 years, many of the treatments written for drugs and reduction of antibiotics [7].

CONSENT FOR PUBLICATION

Not applicable.

CONFLICT OF INTEREST

The authors declare no conflict of interest, financial or otherwise.

ACKNOWLEDGEMENTS

Declared none.

REFERENCES

[1]   Church DL, Lloyd T, Larios O, Gregson DB. Evaluation of Simplexa™ Group A Strep Direct Kit compared to Hologic® Group A streptococcal direct assay for the detection of Group A Streptococcus (GAS) in throat swabs. Journal of clinical microbiology 2018; JCM: 01666-17.

[2]   Marshall S. Giving advice on sore throats. Pharm J 2008; 280(7487): 127.

[3]   Teixeira Rodrigues A, Roque F, Falcão A, Figueiras A, Herdeiro MT. Understanding physician antibiotic prescribing behaviour: a systematic review of qualitative studies. Int J Antimicrob Agents 2013; 41(3): 203-12.
[http://dx.doi.org/10.1016/j.ijantimicag.2012.09.003] [PMID: 23127482]

[4]   NICE CfCPa. Respiratory tract infections-antibiotic prescribing: prescribing of antibiotics for self-limiting respiratory tract infections in adults and children in primary care 2008.

[5]   Baillie L. An exploration of nurse-patient relationships in accident and emergency. Accid Emerg Nurs 2005; 13(1): 9-14.
[http://dx.doi.org/10.1016/j.aaen.2004.10.015] [PMID: 15649681]

[6]   Felsenstein S, Faddoul D, Sposto R, Batoon K, Polanco CM, Dien Bard J. Molecular and clinical diagnosis of group A streptococcal pharyngitis in children. J Clin Microbiol 2014; 52(11): 3884-9.
[http://dx.doi.org/10.1128/JCM.01489-14] [PMID: 25143573]

[7]   Pritt BS, Patel R, Kirn TJ, Thomson RB Jr. Point-counterpoint: a nucleic acid amplification test for *streptococcus pyogenes* should replace antigen detection and culture for the detection of bacterial pharyngitis. J Clin Microbiol 2016; 54(10): 2413-9.
[http://dx.doi.org/10.1128/JCM.01472-16] [PMID: 27440817]

CHAPTER 20

Gonorrhea: *Neisseria Gonorrhoeae* is the Causative Agent

Muhammad Imran Qadir[*] and **Maria Rizvi**

Institute of Molecular Biology & Biotechnology, Bahauddin Zakariya University, Multan, Pakistan

Abstract: Gonorrhea is the 2nd most sexually transmitted disease and is very contagious. The causative agent of this disease is *Neisseria gonorrhoeae.* According to WHO (World Health Organization), the ratio of new cases of gonorrhea reported every year is 1.6 million worldwide. Symptoms of gonorrhea in females are dysuria, vaginal discharge, rectal and/or lower abdominal discomfort, abnormal uterine bleeding, and dyspareunia, and in males, symptoms are dysuria, urethral itch and/or discharge and rectal or testicular pain. Gonorrhea screening is facilitated by NAATs (Nucleic Acid Amplification Tests) in the last decade. Prescribed medication for gonorrhea disease is combination therapy together with a single dosage of ceftriaxone 250 mg given deep into the muscles plus oral intake of either 100 milligrams of doxycycline or 1 gm of azithromycin twice a day for one week. This disease can be prevented by avoiding sexual intercourse, the use of condoms, modifications in sexual practices, and reduction in the number of sex partners.

Keywords: Gonorrhea, NAAT, Sexually Transmitted Disease (STD), Symptoms, Treatment.

INTRODUCTION

Gonorrhea is the set of various clinical conditions in which infection is caused by bacteria acquired sexually [1]. Gonorrhea caused by the bacterium *Neisseria gonorrhoeae* is the 2nd most sexually transmitted infection (STI) and is a very contagious disease that can be transmitted by anal and genital sex and can also be transmitted by oral sex, but less frequently [2]. It has been estimated by WHO worldwide, that 106 million new cases of gonorrhea are reported every year [3]. Gonorrhea affects ethnic, racial, and sexual minorities disproportionately [4]. In certain geographic areas and demographic groups, there have been observed continuously increasing gonorrhea rates. Particularly, 337.5 cases in adolescents,

[*] **Corresponding author Muhammad Imran Qadir:** Institute of Molecular Biology and Biotechnology, Bahauddin Zakariya University, Multan, Pakistan; Tel: +92-61-9210071; Ext. 1920; Fax: +92-61-9210068; E-mail: mrimranqadir@hotmail.com

Muhammad Imran Qadir (Ed.)
All rights reserved-© 2020 Bentham Science Publishers

500.5 cases in adults, 426.6 cases in non-Hispanic blacks, and 128.6 cases in residents of Southern US per 100,000, population are bearing the highest-burden of gonorrhea [5]. Some factors increase the risk of infection such as affected with gonorrhea previously or with other sexually transmitted diseases, age less than twenty-five years, inconsistent use of condoms, having new or many sex partners, using drugs or living in regions where the disease is highly prevalent and commercial sex work [6].

SYMPTOMS

Gonorrhea has symptoms in males and in females it is asymptomatic. Clinical presentations of gonorrhea in females when it is symptomatic include dysuria, vaginal discharge, rectal and/or lower abdominal discomfort, abnormal uterine bleeding, and dyspareunia. Symptoms for males include dysuria, urethral itch, and/or discharge and rectal or testicular pain. The most frequently affected sites of gonorrhea are the cervix and urethra followed by pharyngeal and anal areas [7].

DIAGNOSIS

Gonococcal infections can be prevented in infants by the screening of all women that are sexually active and have a greater risk of infection. Heterosexual women and men who are at low risk for gonorrhea infection are not recommended for screening. Routine screening of gonococcal at anatomical sites of gonorrhea exposure is suggested for sexually active men having sex with men (MSM) every year [6]. Three ways are used to facilitate the diagnosis of gonorrheas such as traditional culture, nucleic acid hybridization, and nucleic acid amplification tests. Traditional culture technology is the only way that is approved to detect *N. gonorrh*ea from both non-genital (conjunctival, pharyngeal, and anorectal) and genital (urethral and endocervical) mucosal surfaces and this technique requires actual cells collected from infected mucosal areas. Cultures may give results of antimicrobial susceptibility and in cases of documented or suspected treatment failure; the cultures ought to be the test of choice. A nucleic acid hybridization test is used in the detection of gonococcal DNA and some of its categories are used for testing chlamydial DNA. These tests are prescribed on samples collected from surfaces of the genital tract such as the vagina and urine. Recently, NAAT is the standard way of screening gonorrhea. Polymerase chain reactions, strand displacement amplification, and transcription-mediated amplification are three basic types of NAATs and to enhance the detection, these types of NAATs identify and then copy gonococcal DNA [1]. This test is usable in both urethral swabs and urine specimens. As compared to culture techniques, NAATs are not much labor-intensive, have improved sensitivity, and have fewer transport requirements and less tight handling [8].

MANAGEMENT

After the development of antibiotic therapy for *Neisseria gonorrhoeae*, the bacteria have developed resistance against the previously used drugs for its treatment, such as penicillin, fluoroquinolones, tetracyclines, and sulfonamides [9]. Medication prescribed for pharyngeal, urogenital and anorectal gonorrhea is combination therapy together with a single dosage of ceftriaxone 250 mg given deep into the muscles plus oral intake of either 100 milligrams of doxycycline or 1 gm of azithromycin twice a day for one week. Prolonged therapy is required in invasive gonorrhea infection (meningitis or endocarditis). If signs remain, sensitivity tests and gonococcal culture tests should be carried out because of having the capability for antibiotic resistance and a specialist of infectious diseases should essentially be consulted. Hospitalization can be required if the infection becomes complicated. For minimal risk of infection again, sexual contact should be avoided at least for a week by patients and until all sex partners are treated. Prevention is important for the individual patient and in communities to improve reproductive and sexual health. Effective strategies for prevention are prior diagnosis, efficient cure, and urge for managing sex partners. Counseling and education are necessary to reduce the infection rate for persons who are at risk and for the asymptomatic gonorrhea infection. After several months of appropriate treatment, retesting for gonorrhea is necessary to detect if the infection is repeated. The behavior for reducing infection rate includes avoiding sexual intercourse, the use of condoms, modifications in sexual practices, and reduction in the number of sex partners [6].

CONSENT FOR PUBLICATION

Not applicable.

CONFLICT OF INTEREST

The authors declare no conflict of interest, financial or otherwise.

ACKNOWLEDGEMENTS

Declared none.

REFERENCES

[1]   Walker CK, Sweet RL. Gonorrhea infection in women: prevalence, effects, screening, and management. Int J Womens Health 2011; 3: 197-206.
[PMID: 21845064]

[2]   Bautista CT, Wurapa E, Sateren WB, Morris S, Hollingsworth B, Sanchez JL. Bacterial vaginosis: a synthesis of the literature on etiology, prevalence, risk factors, and relationship with chlamydia and gonorrhea infections. Mil Med Res 2016; 3(1): 4.

[http://dx.doi.org/10.1186/s40779-016-0074-5] [PMID: 26877884]

[3]   Craig AP, Gray RT, Edwards JL, *et al.* The potential impact of vaccination on the prevalence of gonorrhea. Vaccine 2015; 33(36): 4520-5.
[http://dx.doi.org/10.1016/j.vaccine.2015.07.015] [PMID: 26192351]

[4]   Kirkcaldy RD, Bolan GA, Wasserheit JN. Cephalosporin-resistant gonorrhea in North America. JAMA 2013; 309(2): 185-7.
[http://dx.doi.org/10.1001/jama.2012.205107] [PMID: 23299612]

[5]   Kidd S, Workowski KA. Management of gonorrhea in adolescents and adults in the United States. Clinical Infectious Diseases 2015; 61(suppl_8): S785-801.
[http://dx.doi.org/10.1093/cid/civ731]

[6]   Workowski K. In the clinic. Chlamydia and gonorrhea. Ann Intern Med 2013; 158(3): ITC2-1.
[http://dx.doi.org/10.7326/0003-4819-158-3-201302050-01002] [PMID: 23381058]

[7]   Piszczek J, St. Jean R, Khaliq Y. Treatment update for an increasingly resistant organism. Canadian Pharmacists Journal/Revue des pharmaciens du Canada 2015; 148(2): 9-82.

[8]   Patton ME, Kidd S, Llata E, *et al.* Extragenital gonorrhea and chlamydia testing and infection among men who have sex with men--STD Surveillance Network, United States, 2010-2012. Clin Infect Dis 2014; 58(11): 1564-70.
[http://dx.doi.org/10.1093/cid/ciu184] [PMID: 24647015]

[9]   Stoltey JE, Barry PM. The use of cephalosporins for gonorrhea: an update on the rising problem of resistance. Expert Opin Pharmacother 2012; 13(10): 1411-20.
[http://dx.doi.org/10.1517/14656566.2012.690396] [PMID: 22646654]

CHAPTER 21

Chlamydia: A Common Sexually Transmitted Disease

Muhammad Imran Qadir[*] and **Saba Ghafoor**

Institute of Molecular Biology & Biotechnology, Bahauddin Zakariya University, Multan, Pakistan

Abstract: There are many species of genus *Chlamydia* which causes human diseases, but this genus causing diseases in humans like as *Chlamydia trachomatis* and other species are *C. pneumoniae* that is a human pathogen, *C. psittaci* causes psittacosis in avian but causes infection in humans as zoonosis case, the transmission is rare in-person to person transfer. In women, this leads to severe genital infections like pelvic inflammatory disease, tubal infertility, infertility, ectopic pregnancy, and chronic pelvic pain. The high risk of this infection is usually at a young age. Symptoms are; the burning sensation while urinating or abnormal vaginal discharge, lower abdominal pain, nausea, lower back pain, pain during sex, fever, and pain while passing urine,*etc.* Different types of tests are used to diagnose the infection. Prevention for reduces infection, the use of a condom, number of sex partners will be limited, going to the laboratory regularly for screening. Medicines that are taking against infection are quinolone and tetracycline, erythromycin, clarithromycin, ampicillin, *etc.*

Keywords: Antibiotics, CFT, Culture, PCR, Prevention, Serology, Sexually Transmitted Disease.

INTRODUCTION

There are many species of genus *Chlamydia* which causes human diseases, this genus causing diseases in humans like as *Chlamydia trachomatis* and other species is *C. pneumoniae* that is a human pathogen, *C. psittaci* causes psittacosis in avian but causes infection in humans as zoonosis case, the transmission is rare in-person to person transfer. Chlamydia is caused by bacteria named *Chlamydia trachomatis*. Chlamydia is a bacterial infection that is commonly found all over the world and is sexually transmitted among persons [1]. In women, this leads to severe genital infections like pelvic inflammatory disease, tubal infertility, chronic pelvic pain infertility, and ectopic pregnancy [2]. Due to this, control effort

[*] **Corresponding author Muhammad Imran Qadir:** Institute of Molecular Biology and Biotechnology, Bahauddin Zakariya University, Multan, Pakistan; Tel: +92-61-9210071; Ext. 1920; Fax: +92-61-9210068; E-mail: mrimranqadir@hotmail.com

Muhammad Imran Qadir (Ed.)
All rights reserved-© 2020 Bentham Science Publishers

increases in some countries which enhanced treatment and detection of this infection in young women and taking much more coverage [3].

The particle which is responsible for an infection called the elementary body (EB), which attached the host cells and in the body of an organism by endocytosis. By the formation of the endosome, it enters within the cell and still there in the whole cycle. After 6-8 hours the EB cells changed into a reticulate body (RB) Fig. (**8**). This shows that the organism is active and starts reproduction. The RB is not causing infection. Approximately 48 hours it remains in the cycle and divides through binary fission. Within 24-48 hours some RB cells reorganize into EB and start causing infection. At last, the cells burst, and EB exit from the host cells for the infection in new host cells. Approximately 48 hours take to complete the cycle for virulent lymphogranuloma venereum biovar and trachoma biovar takes 72-96 hours [4]. These are the two strains of C. trachomatis which are divided into two biovars. Diseases caused at mucous membranes and where such types of cells are present by trachoma biovar. Such sites include a conjunctive, endocervical canal, urethra, gastrointestinal, respiratory tracts, and fallopian tubes [5].

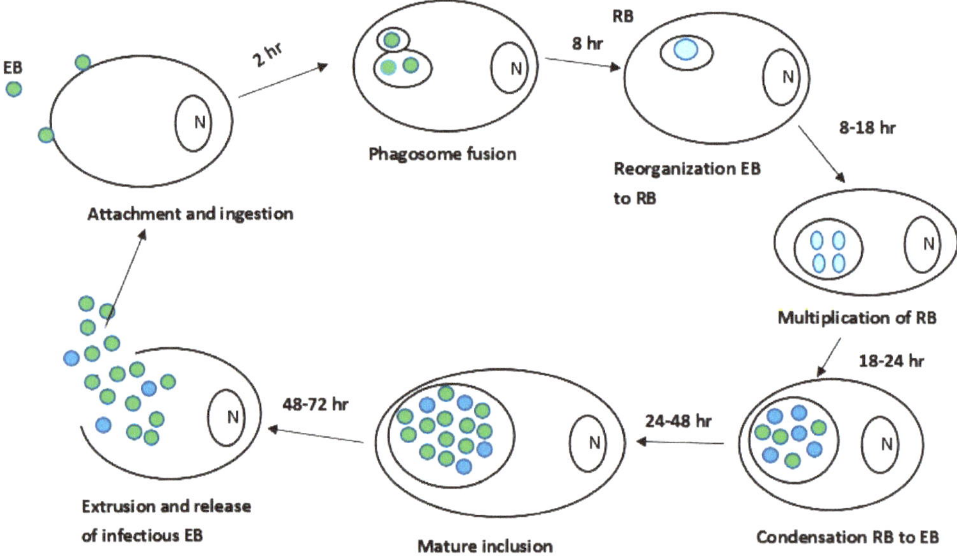

Fig. (8). *Chlamydia trachomatis* and *Chlamydia pneumoniae* infection in human. EB: Elementary body, RB: Reticulate body.

The prevalence of chlamydial infection is most commonly found in sexually active teenagers. The high risk of this infection is usually at a young age [6, 7]. Infants 60%-70% mostly exposed to *C. trachomatis* by passing through the infected birth canal, cause infection. The lymphogranuloma venereum was considered as a disease which causes inguinal buboes and genital ulcer in men. This occurs in such men who have sex with men. For several decades, this circulation is present in the gay community. In endemic areas, this is spread from child to child. In the past, many hundreds of millions were at a high-risk factor for trachoma and millions are blinded. The disease must be disappeared by the improvement of sanitation conditions and all the environmental conditions. In developing countries, it is still a big problem which leads to infectious disease, causing blindness. Children develop infection earlier in holoendemic areas. At adult age, the blindness is caused [4].

SYMPTOMS

Chlamydia is commonly known as the silent disease because of the majority of the females and half of the males having no symptoms. If the symptoms will occur, then it will be within 1-3 weeks after exposure from the virus. Likely symptoms areas; the burning sensation while urinating or abnormal vaginal discharge, lower abdominal pain, nausea, lower back pain, pain during sex, fever, pain while passing urine, bleeding between the menstrual period, frequency passing urine, and a pussy yellowish inflammation of the cervix seen on examination. This infection is not early diagnosed until it becomes complicated. It may cause proctitis which is an infection of rectum lining which will cause sex having a chlamydial partner. In pregnant women this infection causing premature delivery, due to this birth baby having eye infection called conjunctivitis or as pink eye another as pneumonia. In conjunctivitis infection, some type of discharge is excreting from the eyes of the baby and with swollen eyelids in the first 10 days after birth. In pneumonia, it starts with a cough which going to worse condition day by day and congestion in 3-6 weeks after birth. The symptoms shown in men are as discharge from the penis, burning, burning sensation while passing urine, and swelling in the scrotum. This shows the sign of epididymitis (inflammation caused in the male reproductive part). It shows the results of infertility [8].

DIAGNOSIS

Serology

The most common method of diagnosing chlamydia infection is the CFT in the United Kingdom. The micro-immunofluorescence test should be taken for the differentiation between the two species of chlamydia *C. psittaci* and *C. pneumonia* as a complete cell inclusion test of immunofluorescence.

Culture

Cell culture can be used for the chlamydial species. Extreme care should be done in the samples of respiration as in *C. psittaci.* The species of *C. pneumonia* is most problematic for the growing.

Antigen Detection

Antigen detection methods should be used in the diagnosis of ocular infection adults' genital & neonatal infection of *C. trachomatis.* Sputum samples can be detected chlamydia in some commercial assays.

PCR

PCR technique should be used for the diagnosis of respiratory chlamydial infection perfectly because some difficulties occur in the serology results and it resembles the culture of *C. pneumoniae.*

Antibody Detection

There are many methods for the detection of *C. pneumoniae* antibodies in the serum of humans. For patients of all ages the detection of rising titre of IgG is a very suitable method. For younger patients, the detection of IgM is a very suitable method. In older patients, the IgM is less found.

CFT

CFT is the main routine in the laboratory for the pneumonia infection diagnosis. This method cannot be used for the detection of antibodies after the onset of symptoms and also not used for the culture-positive patients to develop CF antibody or absolute increase in titer. It is difficult to find the significance of CFT titers which was taken from the serum's single sample [8].

MANAGEMENT

There are many ways to reduce the risk of spreading infection given below: use condoms while sexual intercourse, the number of sex partners will be limited, going to the laboratory regularly for screening.

The medicines used for the *Chlamydia pneumonia* for *in vitro* susceptibility to macrolide, quinolone and tetracycline antibiotics are used. In the first culture of the lowest MICs erythromycin, clarithromycin and tetracycline should be used. In the second pass, azithromycin should be used at the lowest concentration [9].

The medicines used against *Chlamydia trachomatis* are rifamycin, rifamide, DL473, and rifampin. The combination of the antibiotics tetracycline, erythromycin, or ampicillin with DL473 or rifampin neither be antagonistic nor be synergistic against chlamydia. This type of combination becomes useful for chlamydial infections therapy [10].

CONSENT FOR PUBLICATION

Not applicable.

CONFLICT OF INTEREST

The authors declare no conflict of interest, financial or otherwise.

ACKNOWLEDGEMENTS

Declared none.

REFERENCES

[1]   Organization WH, Organization WH. Global prevalence and incidence of selected curable sexually transmitted infections Overview and estimates Geneva. WHO 2001.

[2]   Stamm WE. *Chlamydia trachomatis* infections of the adult. Sex Transm Dis 1999.

[3]   Gottlieb SL, Brunham RC, Byrne GI, Martin DH, Xu F, Berman SM. The natural history and immunobiology of *Chlamydia trachomatis* genital infection and implications for chlamydia control The Journal of infectious diseases 2010; 201(Supplement_2): s7-s85.

[4]   Schachter J, Stamm W. Chlamydia trachomatis International perspectives on neglected STD's. New York: McGraw-Hill Book Co 1983; pp. 7-35.

[5]   Alary M, Joly JR, Moutquin JM, *et al.* Randomised comparison of amoxycillin and erythromycin in treatment of genital chlamydial infection in pregnancy. Lancet 1994; 344(8935): 1461-5.
       [http://dx.doi.org/10.1016/S0140-6736(94)90288-7] [PMID: 7968119]

[6]   Hillis SD, Nakashima A, Amsterdam L, *et al.* The impact of a comprehensive chlamydia prevention program in Wisconsin. Fam Plann Perspect 1995; 27(3): 108-11.
       [http://dx.doi.org/10.2307/2136107] [PMID: 7672100]

[7]   Donovan P. Testing positive: sexually transmitted disease and the public health response. 1993.

[8]   Adetunde I, Koduah M, Amporful J, Dwummoh–Sarpong A, Nyarko P, Ennin C, *et al.* Epidemiology of Chlamydia Bacteria Infections-A Review. J Am Sci 2009; 5(4): 55-64.

[9]   Kuo C-C, Jackson LA, Lee A, Grayston JT. *In vitro* activities of azithromycin, clarithromycin, and other antibiotics against *Chlamydia pneumoniae*. Antimicrob Agents Chemother 1996; 40(11): 2669-70.
       [http://dx.doi.org/10.1128/AAC.40.11.2669] [PMID: 8913488]

[10]   Jones RB, Ridgway GL, Boulding S, Hunley KL. *In vitro* activity of rifamycins alone and combination with other antibiotics against *Chlamydia trachomatis*. 1983.
       [http://dx.doi.org/10.1093/clinids/5.Supplement_3.S556]

CHAPTER 22

Typhoid Fever: *Salmonella* is the Causative Agent

Muhammad Imran Qadir[*] and **Ayesha Altaf**

Institute of Molecular Biology & Biotechnology, Bahauddin Zakariya University, Multan, Pakistan

Abstract: Typhoid fever which is the systemic disease is caused by the *Salmonella* enterica or *S. typhi*. It has been a disease prevailing throughout the world most common in developing countries, with common symptoms like high fever, constipation, diarrhea, fatigue, and dry cough strategies for its diagnosis have been developed which includes Widal and typhidot, the typhidot technique has advantage on the widal test based on easiness and sensitivity, the different type of antibiotics has been produced for the treatment, but as the bacterial species are becoming resistance there is need for the development of other technique for the treatment which involves the development of vaccines for the prevention of typhoid fever.

Keywords: Antibiotics and Vaccines, High Fever, *Salmonella* enterica, Typhidot, Typhoid, Widal Test.

INTRODUCTION

Salmonella enterica serovar typhi, a gram-negative bacteria is the cause of a disease named typhoid fever or enteric fever which is a systemic disease [1, 2], this disease has challenged humans throughout history and still, it's been a major challenge faced by humans, the host of this bacterium is only human [3]. The various factor contributing to typhoid fever are poor sewerage systems, poor sanitation, and overpopulation [4]. The signs and symptoms of typhoid are high-grade fever, diarrhea, rose spots, and loss of appetite [5].

Although Typhoid is prevalent throughout the world, it is more common in developing countries, in Pakistan it is the sixth most common cause of death, it was estimated in 2000 that about 21 million people throughout the world suffer from typhoid and 0.21 million deaths are caused by it [5].

[*] **Corresponding author Muhammad Imran Qadir:** Institute of Molecular Biology and Biotechnology, Bahauddin Zakariya University, Multan, Pakistan; Tel: +92-61-9210071; Ext. 1920; Fax: +92-61-9210068; E-mail: mrimranqadir@hotmail.com

Muhammad Imran Qadir (Ed.)
All rights reserved-© 2020 Bentham Science Publishers

SYMPTOMS

Typhoid is caused by *S. typhi*, the incubation time of the bacterium is 1-2 weeks and can increase from 3 - 60   days the   illness presents sustained fever and other symptoms which may include abdominal pain, constipation, diarrhea, fatigue, and dry cough [1] and rose spots [2, 6].

DIAGNOSIS

Typhoid fever which is a systemic disease is diagnosed by the Widal test which is widely used for its diagnosis, the test is easy to perform and requires low sophisticated equipment's and minimal training it depends on the agglutination reaction between S.typhi, the flagellar H antigen and somatic Lipopolysaccharides O antigen, one of the disadvantages is that different bacterium has similar properties that's why clinical signs and symptoms of typhoid are not recognized by the Widal test and it may lead patients to receive inappropriate and unnecessary treatment [7, 8]. An alternative strategy for diagnosis is typhidot which is highly sensitive and can easily be performed [9].

MANAGEMENT

As typhoid is an important cause of illness and death its management is important, different types of antibiotics are used for the treatment, for example, chloramphenicol is an antibiotic used for treatment as the bacterial species are becoming resistant to these antibiotics and various other antibiotics like fluoroquinolones, besides, another drug named azithromycin which is effective against multidrug resistance strains is being used, these multidrug resistance strains may lead to severe disease, therefore there is a need to prevent resistance development in strains against antibiotics and to discover new therapies for these salmonelloses [10]. Other managements were made which includes the development of vaccines for the control of typhoid fever, the commercially available vaccines are Ty21a and Vi polysaccharide but these are not used routinely, new modified Vi vaccines named as Vi-eEPA are under development, the disadvantage of these vaccines is these are only used for the *S. typhi*, not for other species other vaccines are under development which are used for the treatment of *Salmonella* species [11, 12].

CONSENT FOR PUBLICATION

Not applicable.

CONFLICT OF INTEREST

The authors declare no conflict of interest, financial or otherwise.

ACKNOWLEDGEMENTS

Declared none.

REFERENCES

[1]   Kabwama SN, Bulage L, Nsubuga F, *et al.* A large and persistent outbreak of typhoid fever caused by consuming contaminated water and street-vended beverages: Kampala, Uganda, January - June 2015. BMC Public Health 2017; 17(1): 23.
[http://dx.doi.org/10.1186/s12889-016-4002-0] [PMID: 28056940]

[2]   Muti M, Gombe N, Tshimanga M, *et al.* Typhoid outbreak investigation in Dzivaresekwa, suburb of Harare City, Zimbabwe, 2011. Pan Afr Med J 2014; 18(1): 309.
[http://dx.doi.org/10.11604/pamj.2014.18.309.4288] [PMID: 25469202]

[3]   Galán JE. Typhoid toxin provides a window into typhoid fever and the biology of *Salmonella* Typhi. Proc Natl Acad Sci USA 2016; 113(23): 6338-44.
[http://dx.doi.org/10.1073/pnas.1606335113] [PMID: 27222578]

[4]   Ayub U, Khattak AA, Saleem A, Javed F, Siddiqui N, Hussain N, *et al.* Incidence of typhoid fever in Islamabad, Pakistan. Am-Eurasian J Toxicol Sci 2015; 7(4): 220-3.

[5]   Tareen AM. Prevalence of typhoid fever in general population of district Quetta, Balochistan, Pakistan. J App Emerg Sci 2016; 5(2): 70-3.

[6]   Humphries RM, Linscott AJ. Laboratory diagnosis of bacterial gastroenteritis. Clin Microbiol Rev 2015; 28(1): 3-31.
[http://dx.doi.org/10.1128/CMR.00073-14] [PMID: 25567220]

[7]   Lalremruata R, Chadha S, Bhalla P. Retrospective audit of the Widal test for diagnosis of typhoid Fever in pediatric patients in an endemic region. J Clin Diagn Res 2014; 8(5): DC22-5.
[PMID: 24995178]

[8]   Wasihun AG, Wlekidan LN, Gebremariam SA, *et al.* Diagnosis and treatment of typhoid fever and associated prevailing drug resistance in northern Ethiopia. Int J Infect Dis 2015; 35: 96-102.
[http://dx.doi.org/10.1016/j.ijid.2015.04.014] [PMID: 25931197]

[9]   Yadav K, Yadav SK, Parihar G. A comparative study of Typhidot and Widal test for rapid diagnosis of typhoid fever. Int J Curr Microbiol Appl Sci 2015; 4(5): 34-8.

[10]   Gal-Mor O, Boyle EC, Grassl GA. Same species, different diseases: how and why typhoidal and non-typhoidal *Salmonella* enterica scrovars differ. Front Microbiol 2014; 5: 391.
[http://dx.doi.org/10.3389/fmicb.2014.00391] [PMID: 25136336]

[11]   Anwar E, Goldberg E, Fraser A, Acosta CJ, Paul M, Leibovici L. Vaccines for preventing typhoid fever. Cochrane Database Syst Rev 2014; (1): CD001261
[PMID: 24385413]

[12]   MacLennan CA, Martin LB, Micoli F. Vaccines against invasive *Salmonella* disease: current status and future directions. Hum Vaccin Immunother 2014; 10(6): 1478-93.
[http://dx.doi.org/10.4161/hv.29054] [PMID: 24804797]

CHAPTER 23

Q Fever: A *Coxiella Burnetii* Infection

Muhammad Imran Qadir[*] and **Adeela Awan**

Institute of Molecular Biology & Biotechnology, Bahauddin Zakariya University, Multan, Pakistan

Abstract: Q fever is a worldwide disease caused by a bacterium *Coxiella burnetti*. The *C. burnetii* is found in goats, sheep, and cows. A higher risk of Q fever is observed in farmers and veterinarians. Acute and chronic diseases are two forms of Q fever. The symptoms of an acute form of Q fever are illness, headache, myalgia, chills, fatigue, sweats, pneumonia, hepatitis, while endocarditis is the most lethal type of chronic form of Q fever. Nucleic acid testing and serological methods are the methods used to diagnose Q fever. In the case of acute disease, an antibiotic Doxycycline (100 mg) is recommended twice a day for its treatment while for endocarditis a combination of doxycycline and hydroxychloroquine or a combination of doxycycline plus a fluoroquinolone (FQ) may be prescribed.

Keywords: Acute and Chronic, *Coxiella burnetii*, Doxycycline, Fluoroquinolones and Endocarditis, Hydroxychloroquine.

INTRODUCTION

Query fever (Q fever) is a worldwide common infectious disease caused by the intracellular, gram-negative, and obligates bacterial form called *Coxiella burnetti*. *C. burnetti* is a bacterial type which is extremely resistant to ecological situations as they form common spores and transmit the infection from animals to humans [1].

PREVALENCE

The Q fever prevalence is observed worldwide but it is not reported in New Zealand. Its prevalence is observed greater in France and Australia as compared to the USA. In the case of age and gender, Q fever is reported in men with age group 40 and 69 because they have to work with animals as compared to women and children [2].

---

[*] **Corresponding author Muhammad Imran Qadir:** Institute of Molecular Biology and Biotechnology, Bahauddin Zakariya University, Multan, Pakistan; Tel: +92-61-9210071; Ext. 1920; Fax: +92-61-9210068; E-mail: mrimranqadir@hotmail.com

Muhammad Imran Qadir (Ed.)
All rights reserved-© 2020 Bentham Science Publishers

CAUSES OF Q FEVER

C. burnetii are the microbes that are typically found in animals such as goats, sheep, cows, ticks, birds, and humans [3]. Humans are infected with Q fever when these animals transmit *C. burnetti* in milk, feces, urine, and fluids from giving birth Fig. (**9**). These substances may be arid in a farmyard where infected dust particles are present in the air. When the humans inhale the impure air, they get an infection of Q fever. In some cases, when humans drink unpasteurized milk, they also get an infection from this source. The higher risk of acquiring Q fever is observed in veterinarians, farmers, people who live close to a farm, researchers in the laboratory of *C. burnetti,* and workers in the meat and dairy industry. In the tase of human contact, the less risk is observed [4].

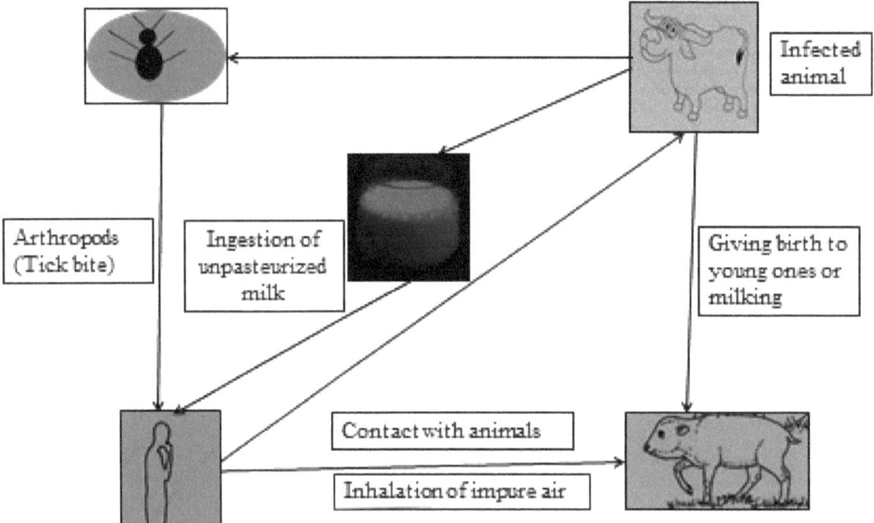

Fig. (9). Transmission of Q fever.

FORMS OF Q FEVER

There are two forms of Q fever:

- Acute Q fever
- Chronic Q fever

Acute Q Fever

The uncommon and less lethal form of Q fever called acute fever develops an incubation period ranging from 2 to 6 weeks. In acute fever cases, most of the patients are asymptomatic while fewer patients may have a mild infection.

Symptoms of Acute Q Fever

The important symptoms in case of acute Q fever are febrile illness, headache, myalgia, chills, fatigue, sweats, Pneumonia, Hepatitis, nausea and vomiting, diarrhea [5].

Chronic Q Fever

The most serious, lethal, and less common type of disease is called chronic Q fever. Patients infected with chronic Q fever may retain this disease from months to years after initial symptoms.

Symptoms of Chronic Q Fever

The main clinical presentation of chronic fever is the inflammation of the inner lining of the heart called endocarditis leading to failure of the heart [6]. The other complications may be inflammation of the central nervous system called encephalitis, the inflammation of the lungs called pneumonia, inflammation of the liver called hepatitis, and infection of bones known as osteomyelitis. The people have weakened the immune system, valvular abnormalities and vascular infections are at high risk for developing chronic fever [7]. Moreover, women during pregnancy are also susceptible to chronic fever and cause miscarriage, low birth weight, premature birth, and stillbirth [8].

DIAGNOSIS

A blood culture diagnoses Q fever. Initially, the nucleic acid testing is performed for the diagnosis of *C. burnetti* through the Polymerase chain reaction (PCR) within a week [8]. But the most preferable method or the diagnosis of *C. burnetii* is Serologic methods. In the serologic method, the detection of phase I and II antibodies IgG titer of 800 or greater against phase I antibodies indicates a chronic infection and A titer of 200 or greater for IgG and 50 or greater for IgM against phase II antibodies indicates recent infection [9].

TREATMENT

100 mg Doxycycline twice daily for 14 days is recommended for adults in case of acute form. In the case of chronic disease, endocarditis is the most serious form and it is recommended that during 2.5 years patients should be treated with a combination of doxycycline and hydroxychloroquine [10]. Nowadays it is recommended that 100 mg two times a day of oral doxycycline and 200mg 3 times a day of hydroxychloroquine is a standard treatment and must be continued

for 18 months. A combination of doxycycline plus a fluoroquinolone (FQ) is recommended for 3-4 years to patients if hydroxychloroquine is not suitable for them [11].

Vaccination is another effective and safe method for treatment against *C. burnetti* and before vaccination; serology testing must be performed to test for cellular immunity [7].

PREVENTION

The risk of exposure to Q fever can be minimized by following precautions [12].

1. Do not drink unpasteurized milk.
2. Clean the place of animals where they are kept.
3. Wash your hands properly with soap and change your clothes after working with animals.
4. The exposed area must be decontaminated properly.
5. The persons working with animals must get the vaccination.
6. The airflow in farmyards must be restricted.
7. Use a respirator when working with animals.

CONSENT FOR PUBLICATION

Not applicable.

CONFLICT OF INTEREST

The authors declare no conflict of interest, financial or otherwise.

ACKNOWLEDGEMENTS

Declared none.

REFERENCES

[1]   Burnet FM, Freeman M. Experimental studies on the virus of "Q" fever. Rev Infect Dis 1983; 5(4): 800-8.
       [http://dx.doi.org/10.1093/clinids/5.4.800] [PMID: 6194551]

[2]   Sloan-Gardner TS, Massey PD, Hutchinson P, Knope K, Fearnley E. Trends and risk factors for human Q fever in Australia,1991-2014. Epidemiol Infect 2017; 145(4): 787-95.
       [http://dx.doi.org/10.1017/S0950268816002843] [PMID: 27927265]

[3]   Raoult D, Marrie T, Mege J. Natural history and pathophysiology of Q fever. Lancet Infect Dis 2005; 5(4): 219-26.
       [http://dx.doi.org/10.1016/S1473-3099(05)70052-9] [PMID: 15792739]

[4]   Parker NR, Barralet JH, Bell AM. Q fever. Lancet 2006; 367(9511): 679-88.
       [http://dx.doi.org/10.1016/S0140-6736(06)68266-4] [PMID: 16503466]

[5]   Karakousis PC, Trucksis M, Dumler JS. Chronic Q fever in the United States. J Clin Microbiol 2006; 44(6): 2283-7.
[http://dx.doi.org/10.1128/JCM.02365-05] [PMID: 16757641]

[6]   Fenollar F, Fournier P-E, Carrieri MP, Habib G, Messana T, Raoult D. Risks factors and prevention of Q fever endocarditis. Clin Infect Dis 2001; 33(3): 312-6.
[http://dx.doi.org/10.1086/321889] [PMID: 11438895]

[7]   Hickie I, Davenport T, Wakefield D, *et al.* Post-infective and chronic fatigue syndromes precipitated by viral and non-viral pathogens: prospective cohort study. BMJ 2006; 333(7568): 575.
[http://dx.doi.org/10.1136/bmj.38933.585764.AE] [PMID: 16950834]

[8]   Fournier P-E, Raoult D. Comparison of PCR and serology assays for early diagnosis of acute Q fever. J Clin Microbiol 2003; 41(11): 5094-8.
[http://dx.doi.org/10.1128/JCM.41.11.5094-5098.2003] [PMID: 14605144]

[9]   Leung-Shea C, Danaher PJ. Q fever in members of the United States armed forces returning from Iraq. Clin Infect Dis 2006; 43(8): e77-82.
[http://dx.doi.org/10.1086/507639] [PMID: 16983603]

[10]   Levy PY, Drancourt M, Etienne J, *et al.* Comparison of different antibiotic regimens for therapy of 32 cases of Q fever endocarditis. Antimicrob Agents Chemother 1991; 35(3): 533-7.
[http://dx.doi.org/10.1128/AAC.35.3.533] [PMID: 2039204]

[11]   Gami AS, Antonios VS, Thompson RL, Chaliki HP, Ammash NM, Eds. Q fever endocarditis in the United States Mayo Clinic Proceedings. Elsevier 2004.

[12]   Lower T, Corben P, Massey P, *et al.* Farmers' knowledge of Q fever and prevention approaches in New South Wales. Aust J Rural Health 2017; 25(5): 306-10.
[http://dx.doi.org/10.1111/ajr.12346] [PMID: 28618042]

CHAPTER 24

Buruli Ulcer: *Mycobacterium Ulcerans* is the Causative Agent

Muhammad Imran Qadir[*] and **Munaza Gilani**

Institute of Molecular Biology & Biotechnology, Bahauddin Zakariya University, Multan, Pakistan

Abstract: Buruli ulcer also called Brainsdale ulcer is the chronic, debilitating subcutaneous destructive infection of the skin, soft tissue, and adipose tissue. *Mycobacterium ulceran*s is the causative agent of BU. The infection of BU is prevalent in many areas of the world. However, wetlands and tropic to sub-tropic areas are more prone. The disease can be diagnosed by expert physicians as it can be confused with the other skin infection.IS2404 PCR is mostly used for the diagnosis of BU. Antibiotics and surgery are frequently used for the treatment. Heat treatment has also been found effective for BU. The condition could lead to disabilities if not treated on time such as amputation of the vital organ *i.e.* eye or the limbs. The affected person may face the problem of social stigma and economic challenges as a consequence of these disabilities. No vaccines are available yet for BU. However, short-lived protection is obtained using the BCG vaccine. The disease is not fatal, however.

Keywords: Deformities, *Mycobacterium ulcerans*, Necrotizing Ulceration, Rifampicin.

INTRODUCTION

Buruli Ulcer (BU) also called the Brainsdale ulcer, has been identified as a re-emerging endemic disease in many countries of the world including Africa, Asia, The Americas, and Western Pacific. But the situation is more dominant in Sub Saharan regions (predominantly in West Africa), where the prevalence of BU is more than tuberculosis [1]. BU has also been reported along the localized coastal area of Victoria in Australia [2]. The wetlands and flooded areas are more prone to BU.

The young adults of less than 15 years are mostly affected by the disease. About 24000 cases had been reported in West African regions (1978-2006), 7000 cases

[*] **Corresponding author Muhammad Imran Qadir:** Institute of Molecular Biology and Biotechnology, Bahauddin Zakariya University, Multan, Pakistan, Tel: +92-61-9210071; Ext. 1920; Fax: +92-61-9210068; E-mail: mrimranqadir@hotmail.com

Muhammad Imran Qadir (Ed.)
All rights reserved-© 2020 Bentham Science Publishers

in Benin (1989-2006), and 21 cases in Nigeria respectively. In Ghana, about 1000 cases are reported annually where the nationwide prevalence is 150.8 / 100,000 individuals. 2037 cases were reported to WHO in 2015. The disease is characterized by chronic, debilitating subcutaneous destructive infection of the skin, soft tissues, and adipose tissue caused by *Mycobacterium ulcerans*, the same potential environmental pathogen which causes leprosy and tuberculosis [3]. The pathogen requires a temperature of 30-32C and low oxygen (2.5%) for its growth. The incubation period for *Mycobacteria ulcerans* is 5-8 weeks. It produces the toxins "mycolactone" which causes tissue damage and suppresses the immune response [4]. The most affected areas are the limbs (forelimbs and hind limbs) where 80% of the infection occurs. In advanced infections, the bones are adversely affected which causes gross disfigurement and deformities. However, the disease is not fatal.

There are controversies about the transmission of the causative agent. Various research projects are underway which will give a better understanding in the future for its dynamic transmission, thus control of the disease. Current studies suggest that the possible mode of transmission of the infection may be the abraded skin or traumatic injuries contaminating water, vegetation, or soil. Non-mammalian vertebrates and invertebrates (snail) have been reported to be the reservoir of *Mycobacteria ulcerans*. The aquatic insects and mosquito could also be a source of transmission of BU [2].

SYMPTOMS

In early infection, the disease appears as a nodule, plaque, papule, or oedema. If left untreated the condition of this ulceration may enlarge with undermined edges. The disease is characterized by a necrotic painless ulcer with no fever. The massive destruction of the skin leads to contracture deformities caused by cytotoxic mycolactone (a potential toxin which causes tissue damage and suppresses the immune response) and macrolide produced by *Mycobacteria ulcerans*. If delayed prolong, the disease may lead to amputation of the affected area, leading to permanent functional disabilities *i.e.* blindness or amputation of limbs.

The affected person may face the problem of social stigma and economic challenges as a consequence of these disabilities.

DIAGNOSIS

Clinical Diagnosis

The disease is diagnosed based on the location of lesions, the extent of pain, geographical area, age, medical and travel history of the patient by the experienced doctors in these endemic areas.

Laboratory Diagnosis

According to WHO guidelines, the disease is diagnosed in the laboratory using IS2404 PCR, biopsy, histopathology, direct microscopy, and culture. However, PCR is most frequently used to test the occurrence of the disease [5]. Early diagnosis and early treatment will ensure the timely recovery from the infection.

DISEASE MANAGEMENT

Medicines

Treatment involves a combination of antibiotics and other complementary treatment irrespective of the stage of infection for 8 weeks [6].

- A combination of rifampicin (10mg/kg once daily)+streptomycin (15mg/kg once daily)
- A combination of rifampicin (10mg/kg once daily) + clarithromycin (7.5mg/kg twice daily) [7]
- A combination of rifampicin (10mg/kg once daily) + moxifloxacin (400mg once daily)

Surgery

Wound management and surgery are performed along with antibiotics to enhance the process of healing [8]. In some cases, surgery is inevitable for treatment in advanced infections. Surgery is performed to remove the necrotic tissue and grafting the resulting defect. Post-surgery nursing care will minimize the duration of treatment. Physiotherapy is performed to prevent the chances of disability in infected persons.

Heat Treatment

Buruli Ulcer can be treated with heat treatment along with sodium acetate trihydrate as a heat application system [9].

Vaccines

Currently, no vaccines are available for Buruli Ulcer [10]. However, short-lived protection is obtained using the BCG vaccine.

Other Preventive Measures

Use of insect repellents, protective clothing, cleaning of skin and wounds after exposure to any contaminated medium, avoiding insect bites and mosquito control can be considered effective for preventing the outbreak of Buruli Ulcer.

CONSENT FOR PUBLICATION

Not applicable.

CONFLICT OF INTEREST

The authors declare no conflict of interest, financial or otherwise.

ACKNOWLEDGEMENTS

Declared none.

REFERENCES

[1]   van der Werf TS, Stienstra Y, Johnson RC, *et al. Mycobacterium ulcerans* disease. Bull World Health Organ 2005; 83(10): 785-91.
        [PMID: 16283056]

[2]   Johnson PD, Lavender CJ. Correlation between Buruli ulcer and vector-borne notifiable diseases, Victoria, Australia. Emerg Infect Dis 2009; 15(4): 614-5.
        [http://dx.doi.org/10.3201/eid1504.081162] [PMID: 19331750]

[3]   Ahorlu CK, Koka E, Yeboah-Manu D, Lamptey I, Ampadu E. Enhancing Buruli ulcer control in Ghana through social interventions: a case study from the Obom sub-district. BMC Public Health 2013; 13(1): 59.
        [http://dx.doi.org/10.1186/1471-2458-13-59] [PMID: 23339623]

[4]   van der Werf TS, Stinear T, Stienstra Y, van der Graaf WT, Small PL. Mycolactones and *Mycobacterium ulcerans* disease. Lancet 2003; 362(9389): 1062-4.
        [http://dx.doi.org/10.1016/S0140-6736(03)14417-0] [PMID: 14522538]

[5]   Phillips R, Horsfield C, Kuijper S, *et al.* Sensitivity of PCR targeting the IS2404 insertion sequence of *Mycobacterium ulcerans* in an Assay using punch biopsy specimens for diagnosis of Buruli ulcer. J Clin Microbiol 2005; 43(8): 3650-6.
        [http://dx.doi.org/10.1128/JCM.43.8.3650-3656.2005] [PMID: 16081892]

[6]   Organization WH. Buruli Ulcer Disease. WHO Fact Sheet No 199 World Health Organization, Geneva, Switzerland 2007. http://www who int/mediacentre/factsheets/fs199/en

[7]   Chauty A, Ardant M-F, Adeye A, *et al.* Promising clinical efficacy of streptomycin-rifampin combination for treatment of buruli ulcer (*Mycobacterium ulcerans* disease). Antimicrob Agents Chemother 2007; 51(11): 4029-35.
        [http://dx.doi.org/10.1128/AAC.00175-07] [PMID: 17526760]

[8]   Asiedu K, Raviglione MC, Scherpbier R. Organization WH, Initiative GBU. Buruli ulcer: *Mycobacterium ulcerans* infection. 2000.

[9]   Junghanss T, Um Boock A, Vogel M, Schuette D, Weinlaeder H, Pluschke G. Phase change material for thermotherapy of Buruli ulcer: A prospective observational single centre proof-of-principle trial. PLoS Negl Trop Dis 2009; 3(2): e380.

[http://dx.doi.org/10.1371/journal.pntd.0000380] [PMID: 19221594]

[10]   Demangel C, Stinear TP, Cole ST. Buruli ulcer: reductive evolution enhances pathogenicity of *Mycobacterium ulcerans*. Nat Rev Microbiol 2009; 7(1): 50-60.
[http://dx.doi.org/10.1038/nrmicro2077] [PMID: 19079352]

CHAPTER 25

Whooping Cough: *Bordetella Pertussis* is the Causative Agent

Muhammad Imran Qadir[*] and **Ramsha Shahzad**

Institute of Molecular Biology & Biotechnology, Bahauddin Zakariya University, Multan, Pakistan

Abstract: Whooping cough is a respiratory tract infection mainly occurs in children and infants. *Bordetella pertussis* is bacteria that is responsible for the cough. It is a gram-negative bacteria that belong to the Cocco-bacillus group. Whooping cough is also known as Pertussis. Parents and siblings play a major role in its transmission. It is transferred from person to person. Illness, sneezing, and cough are the main symptoms. By observing the victim it can diagnose easily, by a blood test or by physical examination. However, the treatment of cough is now present in this era. Vaccination is present for treating pertussis. These vaccines are effective, but not enough efficient in their performance. Before the advent of vaccines, pertussis is an epidemic disease, but nowadays it is working against cough for treatment to some extent. More advanced techniques are trying to discover for treating and curing pertussis.

Keywords: Epidemic, Pertussis, Transmission, Vaccine, Whooping Cough.

INTRODUCTION

Pertussis (whooping cough) is a respiratory tract infection. It is the oldest known epidemic disease. In early times, human beings thought about it had been occurring by an infectious agent like HIV. Later on, the main cause of whooping cough would identify, which is by *Bordetella pertussis*. Before the discovery of vaccination, people thought it was only a childhood disease [1]. It is a gram-negative bacteria that belongs to coccobacillus [2]. *Bordetella pertussis* enters into a respiratory tract which attaches with a cilia line and secret poison, which swells the cilia line and causes cough. It is transmitted by person to person by sneezing mostly by parents and siblings [2, 3]. It can affect all age group people but mostly affects the children or infants badly. It is both endemic and epidemic kind of disease. Vaccines are involved in the treatment of cough. There are different types of vaccines that are used nowadays for the treatment of Pertussis, among different

[*] **Corresponding author Muhammad Imran Qadir:** Institute of Molecular Biology and Biotechnology, Bahauddin Zakariya University, Multan, Pakistan; Tel: +92-61-9210071; Ext. 1920; Fax: +92-61-9210068; E-mail: mrimranqadir@hotmail.com

Muhammad Imran Qadir (Ed.)
All rights reserved-© 2020 Bentham Science Publishers

types of vaccines being used Acellular pertussis is a type of vaccine which is widely used in New Zealand [4]. Babies cannot get vaccination until they reached the age of two months.

SYMPTOMS

Serious illness mainly occurs in infants, children, and somehow in adults but it also occurs sometimes without showing any illness Fig. (**10**).

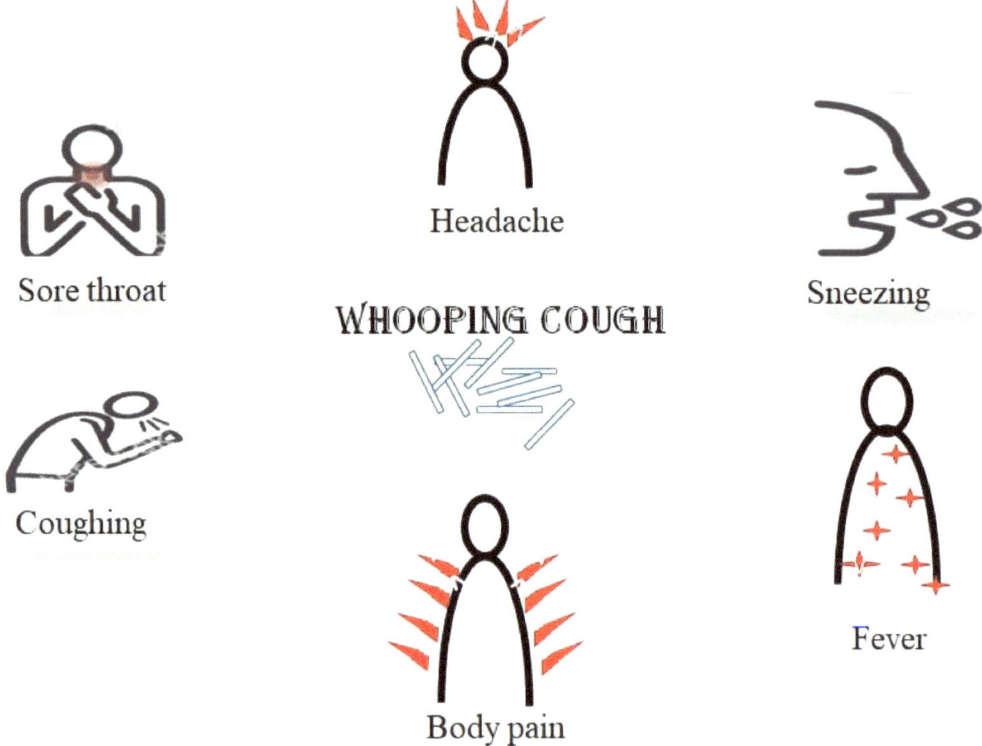

Fig. (10). Symptoms of whooping cough.

Usually, a symptom occurs within 5-15 days after exposure, common symptom includes sneezing, cough, and fever, *etc.* [2, 5].

DIAGNOSIS

By considering the victim, whooping cough is simply diagnosed. Few more steps are also done for diagnoses such as blood tests, symptoms, and physical examination. In recent advances, new techniques are used for diagnosis, especially for those infants who have no vaccination against pertussis like antigen detection by PCR, most sensitive antigen detection into a blood serum and oral fluid. All these techniques have a rapid contribution in diagnosis and for preventing measures [5].

TREATMENT

Mainly treatment is not started in its early stages. In its harsh conditions, treatments are given to the patient from different ways depending on its severity.

Medicines are used to cure pertussis in a form of syrups such as hydryllin, tutsyia, and Benadryl.

Surgery and radiotherapy are not involved in pertussis treatment.

Vaccines are widely used for their curing purpose. For short treatment, erythromycin and azithromycin are used. There are macrolide antibiotics. Antibiotics have no clinical effect on pertussis but it eradicates *B. pertussis* to reduce the spreading infection. Unfortunately, there are still no disease-specific therapies present against pertussis.

Vaccines for Pertussis

From 1926 to 1930, approximately more than 30,000 deaths occurred due to pertussis in the USA. At the time of 1906 few organisms found to be used for vaccination. With early vaccination development, more doses were involved against pertussis treatment. In very early stages of vaccine formation, a whole-cell pertussis vaccine was developed. Later on, acellular vaccines of pertussis were developed. Numbers of proteins or factors were found in pertussis as toxins that were used as vaccines against cough [2]. In recent studies, vitamin C is found to have an efficient effect against whooping cough. Sodium ascorbate is another chemical involved in preventing measures of cough. Acellular vaccines need more doses as quantity increases reduce the efficiency of an immune system against cough. The natural immunity power against whooping cough remains at least 30 years while vaccine immunity remains for 3 years. Liposomal sodium ascorbate obtained from Amazon or i-herb. As vitamin C is non-toxic to a human body, its excess amount is naturally removed from the body even during the treatment of whooping cough. So many works have done by the body with the use of vitamin C [6].

CONSENT FOR PUBLICATION

Not applicable.

CONFLICT OF INTEREST

The authors declare no conflict of interest, financial or otherwise.

ACKNOWLEDGEMENTS

Declared none.

REFERENCES

[1]   Aslanabadi A, Ghabili K, Shad K, Khalili M, Sajadi MM. Emergence of whooping cough: notes from three early epidemics in Persia. Lancet Infect Dis 2015; 15(12): 1480-4.
[http://dx.doi.org/10.1016/S1473-3099(15)00292-3] [PMID: 26298206]

[2]   Cherry JD. The history of pertussis (whooping cough); 1906–2015: facts, myths, and misconceptions. Curr Epidemiol Rep 2015; 2(2): 120-30.
[http://dx.doi.org/10.1007/s40471-015-0041-9]

[3]   Zöldi V, Sane J, Nohynek H, Virkki M, Hannila-Handelberg T, Mertsola J. Decreased incidence of pertussis in young adults after the introduction of booster vaccine in military conscripts: Epidemiological analyses of pertussis in Finland, 1995-2015. Vaccine 2017; 35(39): 5249-55.
[http://dx.doi.org/10.1016/j.vaccine.2017.08.008] [PMID: 28823620]

[4]   Kiedrzynski T, Bissielo A, Suryaprakash M, Bandaranayake D. Whooping cough—where are we now? A review. N Z Med J 2015; 128(1416): 21-7.
[PMID: 26117672]

[5]   Wang K, Bettiol S, Thompson MJ, *et al.* Symptomatic treatment of the cough in whooping cough. Cochrane Database Syst Rev 2014; (9): CD003257
[http://dx.doi.org/10.1002/14651858.CD003257.pub5] [PMID: 25243777]

[6]   Humphries S. Vitamin C Treatment of Whooping Cough–Where Vaccines and Antibiotics Have Failed. Newsletter 2018.

CHAPTER 26

Tetanus (Lockjaw): A *Clostridum Tetani* Infection

Muhammad Imran Qadir[*] and **Iqra Shahzadi**

Institute of Molecular Biology & Biotechnology, Bahauddin Zakariya University, Multan, Pakistan

Abstract: Tetanus is also known as lockjaw, *Clostridium tetani* are its infectious agent. A toxin is produced by that bacteria affects the nervous system and brain, which leads to muscle stiffness. Neurotoxin affects the nerves which control the movement of muscles when the spores of *Clostridium tetani* entered into the wound. When tetanospasmin enters into the bloodstream, it spreads into the body immediately, appearing tetanus symptoms. The person who is suffering from stiffness and muscle swamp should go for the medical checkup instantaneously. After 7 to 10 days of starting infection, the symptoms of tetanus usually appear. Doctors prescribe metronidazole or penicillin for tetanus treatment. These antibiotics stop the bacterium from producing endotoxin and multiplying that causes stiffness of muscles and muscle spasms. Tetracycline is given to allergic patients instead of penicillin and metronidazole.

Keywords: *Clostridium tetani*, Metronidazole, Penicillin, Tetanus, Tetanospasmin, Tetracycline.

INTRODUCTION

Tetanus is a disease caused by bacteria. The bacteria present in manure, environmental agents, and soil. A person who has a wound with polluted objects and got the infection that can damage the whole body [1]. It can be fatal. It is also known as lockjaw, *Clostridium tetani* are its infectious agent. A toxin produced by those bacteria affects the nervous system and brain, which leads to muscle stiffness [2]. Neurotoxin affects the nerves that control the movement of muscles when the spores of *Clostridium tetani* entered into the wound. In America, there are almost thirty cases per year [3]. Many people do not get vaccinated or do not take boosters within 10 years. Tetanus should be medically treated immediately. It will require antibiotics and violent wound treatment [4]. Serious breathing difficulties and muscle spasms caused by this infection which can be dangerous.

[*] **Corresponding author Muhammad Imran Qadir:** Institute of Molecular Biology and Biotechnology, Bahauddin Zakariya University, Multan, Pakistan; Tel: +92-61-9210071; Ext. 1920; Fax: +92-61-9210068; E-mail: mrimranqadir@hotmail.com

Muhammad Imran Qadir (Ed.)
All rights reserved-© 2020 Bentham Science Publishers

The treatment of tetanus is not effected uniformly although it exists. The vaccine is the only method to escape from tetanus [5].

CAUSES

Clostridium tetani bacterium caused tetanus. The spores of this bacterium can live for the long-duration exterior of the body. When it got into the body it increases in number rapidly and produced tetanospasmin that is a neurotoxin [6]. When tetanospasmin enters into the bloodstream, it spreads into the body immediately, symptoms of tetanus appear. Tetanospasmin disrupts the signals coming from the brain to nerves and then the spinal cord, and then towards the muscles, causing muscle stiffness and spasms [6]. Mostly *Clostridium tetani* go inside the body mainly by the skin or through the wounds. If ant cut is cleaned thoroughly then infection is not developed. The easy way to diminishing tetanus is: which includes dead cells, wounds that are polluted with crush injuries, saliva, feces, or burns [5]. The rare methods of diminishing tetanus include injections in the muscle, insect bites, surgical procedures, compound fractures, intravenous drug use, superficial wounds, intravenous drug use, and dental infections.

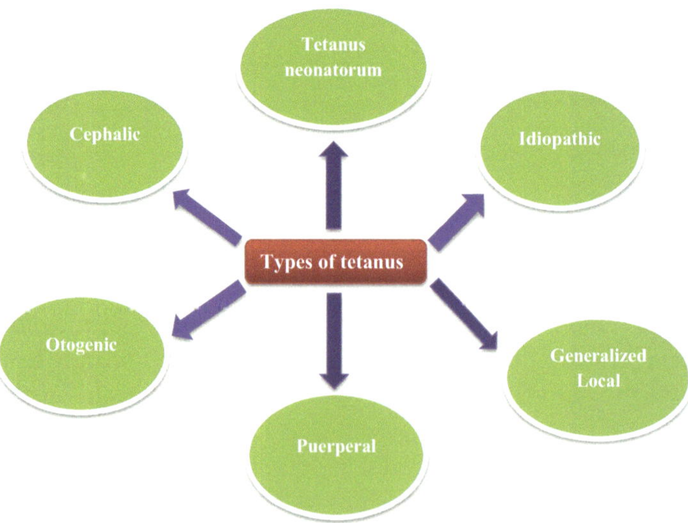

Fig. (11). Types of tetanus.

SYMPTOMS

After 7 to 10 days of starting infection, the symptoms of tetanus usually appear. But it may change from 4 to 21 days and in other cases, it prolonged till months

[7]. Commonly, if the injured place is away from the brain, the incubation period prolonged. If the incubation period is shorter patients have more harsh symptoms. Stiffness and spasms are symptoms of muscles [8]. Stiffness usually began with the grinding of muscles, therefore, called lockjaw. Throat and neck are affected by the muscle swamp and cause problems in swallowing. The spasms of facial muscle have common in patients. The stiffness of the chest and neck muscle may cause breathing difficulties [9]. Limb and abdominal muscles are also influenced by some people. In some cases when the infection is spread to back muscles, the spine roguish backward. It occurs usually when the disease of tetanus occurred in children Fig. (**11**). The symptoms of tetanus in organisms are as followed: rapid heartbeat, headache, bloody stools, sore throat, fever, touch sensitivity, diarrhea, and sweating [7].

DIAGNOSIS

Most doctors never tackled tetanus patients in many areas of the world. Infection is rare because the vaccine against tetanus is mostly given in childhood for immunity. For example, in 2009 in America, only 19 patients of tetanus were found. The treatment is more active when tetanus is analyzed in the early stages. A person who has stiffness and muscle swamp, the tetanus symptoms are more effectively-identified in him [10]. The patient who is taking drugs, the symptoms of tetanus appear later because their medical conditions are different [11]. A blood test confirmed the presence of disease. The person who is suffering from stiffness and muscle swamp should go for the medical checkup instantaneously. The danger of life is greater if the patient is not under the observation of a doctor and the death rate is different from forty to seventy-six percent [9].

COMPLICATIONS MAY COMPRISE

- Fractures Sometimes, bone fractures may lead by muscle convulsions and spasms, in severe cases.
- Pulmonary embolism Blood vessels of the lungs blocked and affect circulation and breathing. The patient will instantly require anti-clotting medication and oxygen therapy.
- Aspiration pneumonia If the stomach's contents and secretions are gasped, lower respiratory tract infections develop, causing pneumonia.
- Tetanic seizures A person who is affected with tetanus experience fits if infection extends to the brain.
- Laryngospasm Spasm of the voice box cause breathing difficulties. The patient may suffocate in severe cases.

TREATMENT

Wounds should be completely cleaned to stop the infection. A tetanus cut or wound must be treated immediately by a professional of medical [12].

A cut or wound which can be developed tetanus is demarcated as:

- A burn or wound which is delayed for over six hours or that needs surgical intervention.
- A burn or wound that comprises a significant quantity of dead tissues.
- Any injury or a wound that has been interacted with soil or manure.
- When the bone is bear to the infection during serious fractures.
- Burns or wounds with systemic sepsis in the patient.

Any patient who has any type of wound listed above may receive tetanus immunoglobulin (TIG) even they have been vaccinated. Immunoglobulin comprises antibodies that destroy *Clostridium tetani* [13]. It protects against tetanus when injected into the vein. TIG does not replace the long term effects on the short term effects of vaccination. TIG injections are safe to administer to pregnant or breastfeeding mothers. Doctors may prescribe metronidazole or penicillin for tetanus treatment. These antibiotics stop the bacterium from producing endotoxin and multiplying that causes stiffness and muscle spasms. Tetracycline is given to allergic patients instead of penicillin and metronidazole [2].

In treating muscle stiffness and spasms, patients may be recommended:

- Diazepam is anticonvulsants, works as a sedative, relax the muscles, prevent spasms, and reduce anxiety [2].
- Baclofen is a muscle relaxant that suppresses nerve signals and resulting in low muscle tension [14].
- A blocking agent such as Neuromuscular blocks the signals from nerves to muscle fibers. It is useful in directing muscle spasms. They include vecuronium and pancuronium [15].

VACCINATION

Tetanus vaccine is regularly given to kids as part of a cellular pertussis shot (DtaP), diphtheria and tetanus toxoids. 5 shots of DTaP vaccine are given in the thighs or the arms of children when they are of 2, 4, 6, 15, or 18 months and 4 to 6 years of age [7]. Between the 11 and 18 years of age, a booster is usually given and then after a decade, another booster is provided. If any person is visiting any area where tetanus is present usually then he should go to a doctor for vaccinations. Tetanus immune globulin may also be provided to the patient in this condition which could stop infection [13]. It is necessary to cure this disease by medical work because after any infection tetanus immune globulin is active for a short time [12].

PREVENTION

The people who are not vaccinated or do not have boosters within the last ten years are affected by tetanus.

CONSENT FOR PUBLICATION

Not applicable.

CONFLICT OF INTEREST

The authors declare no conflict of interest, financial or otherwise.

ACKNOWLEDGEMENTS

Declared none.

REFERENCES

[1]   Brüggemann H, Bäumer S, Fricke WF, *et al.* The genome sequence of Clostridium tetani, the causative agent of tetanus disease. Proc Natl Acad Sci USA 2003; 100(3): 1316-21.
        [http://dx.doi.org/10.1073/pnas.0335853100] [PMID: 12552129]

[2]   Ahmadsyah I, Salim A. Treatment of tetanus: an open study to compare the efficacy of procaine penicillin and metronidazole. Br Med J (Clin Res Ed) 1985; 291(6496): 648-50.
        [http://dx.doi.org/10.1136/bmj.291.6496.648] [PMID: 3928066]

[3]   Pascual FB, McGinley EL, Zanardi LR, Cortese MM, Murphy TV. Tetanus surveillance-United States, 1998-2000. Morbidity and mortality weekly report. MMWR CDC Surveill Summ 2003; 52(3)

[4]   Edmondson RS, Flowers MW. Intensive care in tetanus: management, complications, and mortality in 100 cases. BMJ 1979; 1(6175): 1401-4.
        [http://dx.doi.org/10.1136/bmj.1.6175.1401] [PMID: 445102]

[5]   Simpson L. Botulinum neurotoxin and tetanus toxin. Elsevier 2012.

[6]   Campbell JI, Lam TM, Huynh TL, *et al.* Microbiologic characterization and antimicrobial susceptibility of Clostridium tetani isolated from wounds of patients with clinically diagnosed tetanus. Am J Trop Med Hyg 2009; 80(5): 827-31.
        [http://dx.doi.org/10.4269/ajtmh.2009.80.827] [PMID: 19407132]

[7]   Kretsinger K, Broder KR, Cortese MM, *et al.* Preventing tetanus, diphtheria, and pertussis among adults: use of tetanus toxoid, reduced diphtheria toxoid and acellular pertussis vaccine recommendations of the Advisory Committee on Immunization Practices (ACIP) and recommendation of ACIP, supported by the Healthcare Infection Control Practices Advisory Committee (HICPAC), for use of Tdap among health-care personnel. MMWR Recomm Rep 2006; 55(RR-17): 1-37.
        [PMID: 17167397]

[8]   Rings DM. Clostridial disease associated with neurologic signs: tetanus, botulism, and enterotoxemia. Vet Clin North Am Food Anim Pract 2004; 20(2): 379-391, vii-viii.
[http://dx.doi.org/10.1016/j.cvfa.2004.02.006] [PMID: 15203231]

[9]   Crone NE, Reder AT. Severe tetanus in immunized patients with high anti-tetanus titers. Neurology 1992; 42(4): 761-4.
[http://dx.doi.org/10.1212/WNL.42.4.761] [PMID: 1565228]

[10]   Colombet I, Saguez C, Sanson-Le Pors M-J, Coudert B, Chatellier G, Espinoza P. Diagnosis of tetanus immunization status: multicenter assessment of a rapid biological test. Clin Diagn Lab Immunol 2005; 12(9): 1057-62.
[http://dx.doi.org/10.1128/CDLI.12.9.1057-1062.2005] [PMID: 16148171]

[11]   Abrahamian FM, Pollack CV Jr, LoVecchio F, Nanda R, Carlson RW. Fatal tetanus in a drug abuser with "protective" antitetanus antibodies. J Emerg Med 2000; 18(2): 189-93.
[http://dx.doi.org/10.1016/S0736-4679(99)00192-4] [PMID: 10699520]

[12]   Keller MA, Stiehm ER. Passive immunity in prevention and treatment of infectious diseases. Clin Microbiol Rev 2000; 13(4): 602-14.
[http://dx.doi.org/10.1128/CMR.13.4.602] [PMID: 11023960]

[13]   Kabura L, Ilibagiza D, Menten J, Van den Ende J. Intrathecal *vs* . intramuscular administration of human antitetanus immunoglobulin or equine tetanus antitoxin in the treatment of tetanus: a meta-analysis. Trop Med Int Health 2006; 11(7): 1075-81.
[http://dx.doi.org/10.1111/j.1365-3156.2006.01659.x] [PMID: 16827708]

[14]   Saissy JM, Demazière J, Vitris M, *et al.* Treatment of severe tetanus by intrathecal injections of baclofen without artificial ventilation. Intensive Care Med 1992; 18(4): 241-4.
[http://dx.doi.org/10.1007/BF01709840] [PMID: 1430590]

[15]   Hassel B. Tetanus: pathophysiology, treatment, and the possibility of using botulinum toxin against tetanus-induced rigidity and spasms. Toxins (Basel) 2013; 5(1): 73-83.
[http://dx.doi.org/10.3390/toxins5010073] [PMID: 23299659]

CHAPTER 27

Diphtheria: *Corynebacterium Diphtheria* is the Causative Agent

Muhammad Imran Qadir[*] and **Asma Jan Muhammad**

Institute of Molecular Biology & Biotechnology, Bahauddin Zakariya University, Multan, Pakistan

Abstract: Diphtheria is an acute disease caused by a specific bacterium *Corynebacterium diphtheriae*. In 1883, Klebs first discovered this bacterium in diphtheritic membranes. Diphtheria can spread from one person to another person by direct contact or it may be spread by air. Different symptoms occur during infection and symptoms appear after 7 days of infection. Symptoms of the disease are changed from mild to severe. When the diphtheria disease occurs then a thick covering is formed in the throat. This covering causes difficulty during breathing and it can block the airway. PCR, ICS, and Elek test are used for the diagnosis of the toxin. Mostly children and adult lives are threatening by diphtheria. Vaccines are available for diphtheria disease. 5% to 10% of deaths occur in the affected person. Antibiotics and antitoxin are also available for the treatment of the disease.

Keywords: Antitoxin, Antibiotics, Diphtheria, ICS, Pseudo membrane.

INTRODUCTION

Diphtheria is an acute disease caused by a specific bacterium *Corynebacterium diphtheriae*. In 1883 Klebs first discovered this bacterium in diphtheritic membranes Table **2**. Diphtheria can spread by air, direct contact, and contaminated objects. Diphtheria can also spread with cough and sneezes of an infected person. When the diphtheria disease occurs then a thick covering is formed in the throat. This covering causes difficulty during breathing and it can block the airway. Diphtheria can cause paralysis, heart failure, and may even cause death. The symptoms of Diphtheria disease are changed from mild to severe. The symptoms appear two to five days after infection. In the beginning, the symptoms come gradually with the fever and sore throat but in severe condition, a white layer is formed at the back of the throat [1]. Diphtheria can

[*] **Corresponding author Muhammad Imran Qadir:** Institute of Molecular Biology and Biotechnology, Bahauddin Zakariya University, Multan, Pakistan; Tel: +92-61-9210071; Ext. 1920; Fax: +92-61-9210068; E-mail: mrimranqadir@hotmail.com

Muhammad Imran Qadir (Ed.)
All rights reserved-© 2020 Bentham Science Publishers

spread from one person to another person by direct contact or it may be spread by air. Sometimes *Corynebacterium diphtheriae* is present in some people but they have no sign of disease but they can spread the Diphtheria in other people. Mostly children and adult lives are threatening by diphtheria. Vaccines are available for diphtheria disease [2]. 5% to 10% of deaths occur of the affected person.

Table 2. History of diphtheria.

History	*Work*
5th century BCE	Hippocrates is the first to describe the disease.
6th century	First observations of diphtheria epidemics by the Greek physician Aetius.
1883	The bacteria identified by the German scientists Edwin Klebs and Friedrich Löffler.
1892	Antitoxin treatment, derived from horses, first used in the U.S.
The 1920s	Development of the toxoid used in vaccines

SYMPTOMS

Different symptoms occur during infection and symptoms appear after 7 days of infection. The different signs and symptoms of diphtheria are painful swallowing, headache, cough, sore throat, fatigue, fever, difficulty in breathing, nasal discharge. When infection occurs then healthy tissues are destroyed in the respiratory system [3]. These destroyed tissues form a layer in the throat or nose. This layer is also called a pseudomembrane. This membrane covers the tissues in tonsils, voice box, and nose cause difficulty in breathing [4].

DIAGNOSIS

Different tests are used for the identification of diphtheria. These are the following tests.

ICS Test

ICS test ICS is standing by an immune-chromatographic strip and it is used for the detection of toxin produce by diphtheria [5].

Elek's Test

Elek's test The Elek test is also called an immuno-diffusion technique. This test is used to check the toxigenicity of *C. diphtheriae*. Stephen Dyonis Elek was a microbiologist and discovered the Elek test. An antitoxin paper strip is used in the Elek test [6].

PCR

PCR The PCR is used for the detection of toxin genes present in diphtheria. Specific primers are used for the detection of a toxic gene.

Enzyme Immunoassay (EIA)

Enzyme Immunoassay (EIA) The EIA is another diagnostic test use for the detection and identification of toxigenicity of diphtheria and enzyme immunoassay is a simple, accurate, rapid method. In EIA polyclonal antitoxin is used [7].

MANAGEMENT

When diphtheria infection occurs then different treatments should be taken from the prevention of disease. Antitoxin and antibiotics are administered to neutralize and kill the bacteria and its infection. In the early stage, diphtheria antitoxin should be used to reduce bacterial infection [3].

Diphtheria is a serious disease therefore doctors try to treat it immediately. They recommend an antitoxin and antibody.

Antitoxin

When diphtheria infection occurs then doctors administer an antitoxin to remove and neutralize the toxin that is already present in the bloodstream of an infected person. Doctors perform a different allergy test before administering the antitoxin to make sure that the infected one has not any allergic problem [8].

Antibiotics

Another important element that is used for the treatment of diphtheria is antibiotics which include penicillin or erythromycin. These antibiotics are used to kill the bacteria and remove the infections and the recovery period is a few days after antibiotics taken [9].

Vaccines

Diphtheria vaccines are available that use against *C. diphtheriae.* The vaccine reduces the number of affected people. During childhood, three doses are recommended. Diphtheria vaccine is safe and has no side effects and only a bump is formed at the injection site of the vaccine. The diphtheria vaccine is administered with a combination of other vaccines *e.g.* Hib vaccine and hepatitis vaccine. Infanrix and Daptacel are the brand name of the diphtheria vaccine [9].

Prevention

The infected person should be away from healthy persons. If anyone exposed to an infected person then he must be a visit to the hospital for testing. A person must need a booster dose of the diphtheria vaccine. If a person, especially children, has an infection then must be in the hospital for the proper treatment and should be isolated from another person because diphtheria can spread more frequently from one person to another [10].

CONSENT FOR PUBLICATION

Not applicable.

CONFLICT OF INTEREST

The authors declare no conflict of interest, financial or otherwise.

ACKNOWLEDGEMENTS

Declared none.

REFERENCES

[1]   Drutz E, Edwards MS. Diphtheria, tetanus, and pertussis immunization in infants and children 0 through 6 years of age. UpToDate Retrieved from www.uptodate.com 2020.

[2]   Holý O, Vlčková J, Janoušková L, Matoušková I. Prevalence of diphtheria, tetanus and pertussis in the world. Klinicka mikrobiologie a infekcni lekarstvi 2017; 23(1): 10-6.

[3]   Hoskisson PA. Microbe Profile: *Corynebacterium diphtheriae* - an old foe always ready to seize opportunity. Microbiology 2018; 164(6): 865-7.
[http://dx.doi.org/10.1099/mic.0.000627] [PMID: 29465341]

[4]   Mahomed S, Archary M, Mutevedzi P, *et al.* An isolated outbreak of diphtheria in South Africa, 2015. Epidemiol Infect 2017; 145(10): 2100-8.
[http://dx.doi.org/10.1017/S0950268817000851] [PMID: 28478776]

[5]   James J, Mathews S, Thulaseedharan N. Faucial diphtheria. QJM: An International Journal of Medicine 2017.

[6]   Engler KH, Efstratiou A, Norn D, *et al.* Immunochromatographic strip test for rapid detection of diphtheria toxin: description and multicenter evaluation in areas of low and high prevalence of diphtheria. J Clin Microbiol 2002; 40(1): 80-3.
[http://dx.doi.org/10.1128/JCM.40.1.80-83.2002] [PMID: 11773096]

[7]   Efstratiou A, Engler KH, Mazurova IK, Glushkevich T, Vuopio-Varkila J, Popovic T. Current approaches to the laboratory diagnosis of diphtheria 2000.
[http://dx.doi.org/10.1086/315552]

[8]   Guthrie E, Amirthalingam G. Whooping cough: public health management and guidance. Stroke 2018; 13: 57.

[9]   Organization WH. Diphtheria vaccine: WHO position paper, August 2017 - Recommendations. Vaccine 2018; 36(2): 199-201.
[http://dx.doi.org/10.1016/j.vaccine.2017.08.024] [PMID: 28822645]

[10]   Zanoni G, Zanotti R, Schena D, Sabbadini C, Opri R, Bonadonna P. Vaccination management in children and adults with mastocytosis. Clin Exp Allergy 2017; 47(4): 593-6.
[http://dx.doi.org/10.1111/cea.12882] [PMID: 28079293]

CHAPTER 28

Cholera: A Waterborne Disease Characterized by Diarrhea

Muhammad Imran Qadir[*] and **Azra Yasmeen**

Institute of Molecular Biology & Biotechnology, Bahauddin Zakariya University, Multan, Pakistan

Abstract: Cholera is a disease caused by a bacterial strain *Vibrio cholerae* in the small intestine which is a waterborne disease characterized by diarrhea cause loss of water from the body. *Vibrio cholerae* is the major etiology agent of the cholera disease. There are two O1 and O139 strains of bacteria that produce a toxin which can cause cholera disease, blood infection, and also cause the economic loss of the world. The major causes of cholera are contaminated food and unhygienic water. The bacteria causing the disease exist in water, lakes, and rivers. Over 100,000 deaths occur each year due to cholera. Different management systems are used to control the disease in which different vaccines are used like a rotavirus vaccine, Killed Oral Cholera Vaccine, which includes Dukoral, Shankol, and Euvichol. Different antibiotics used for control of disease and oral-radiation therapy are used to control the disease. Infectious diseases are avoided by taking different preventive measures like hygienic food and hygienic water.

Keywords: Cholera, Cholkit Test, Diarrhea, Dipstick Test, Hygienic Food, Hygienic Water, Rotavirus Vaccine, *Vibrio cholerae*.

INTRODUCTION

Cholera is a disease caused by a bacterial strain *Vibrio cholerae* in the small intestine which is waterborne disease diarrhea that causes loss of water from the body. *Vibrio cholerae* is the major etiology agent of the cholera disease. There are two O1 and O139 strains of bacteria that produce a toxin which can cause cholera disease, blood infection, and also cause the economic loss of the world. It is an infectious disease and the bacterial strain present in contaminated food and water, and this bacterial infection spread due to unhygienic conditions [1]. This bacterial strain is gram-negative. The major cause of cholera is food and water which is contaminated with faces and this problem occurs due to lack of sanitation. So this

[*] **Corresponding author Muhammad Imran Qadir:** Institute of Molecular Biology and Biotechnology, Bahauddin Zakariya University, Multan, Pakistan; Tel: +92 61 9210071, Ext. 1920; Fax: +92-61-9210068; E-mail: mrimranqadir@hotmail.com

Muhammad Imran Qadir (Ed.)
All rights reserved-© 2020 Bentham Science Publishers

bacterial strain gets high prevalence due to the unhygienic food and water uptake [2]. There are different risk factors for cholera which include unhygienic and unboiled water; poverty is one of the factors for cholera, and lack of proper sanitation. And some risk factors related to the food which includes the uptake of specific food products like vegetables, fruits, or rice and consumption of shellfish. And another risk factor is the association between the host and the pathogen *Vibrio cholerae*. These bacteria also found in rivers, lacks, and water coastal. This bacterium affects aquatic animals so industries that are related to these aquatic organisms are also affected. And the contaminated water can cause infection in neighboring areas. There are many outbreaks of cholera in different countries of the world like Kenya, Bangladesh, and Haiti [3]. Over 100,000 deaths occur each year due to cholera disease. The two strains O1 and O139 cause an outbreak in Bangladesh, Kenya [4]. Cholera can spread by drinking contaminated water or food with the feces of the infected person, lack of hygienic conditions, reduced sanitation, and in congested areas. In 2015 due to cholera 28,800 deaths occurred worldwide. Globally cholera spread in 50 countries of the world including Africa, Asia and Karbala, and so on the first outburst of cholera occurred in India in the region of Bengal, then from India, this disease spread in different countries of the world like Asia, Europe. In the past, it was thought that cholera occurred due to contaminated air but scientist Jhon Snow showed that cholera occurred due to contaminated water because the bacterial agent *Vibrio cholerae* lived in water conditions Fig. (**12**), and he proved this statistically during the epidemic of cholera in London in the 19th century [5].

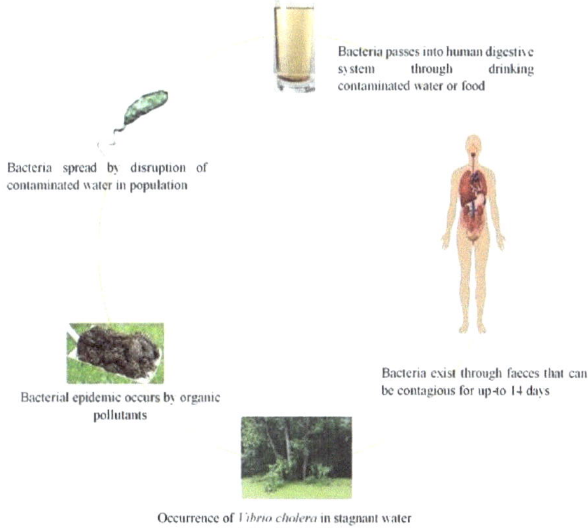

Fig. (12). The life cycle of *Vibrio cholerae*.

SYMPTOMS

Different symptoms appeared during cholera and different tests are used to diagnose cholera and different medicines and vaccines are used to control that disease and some preventive measures are used to prevent the disease. There are some common symptoms and some acute cholera cases. Cholera can cause a large amount of diarrhea which can cause loss of a large amount of water from the body, vomiting, cramping of muscles, and severe conditions that cause dehydration and imbalance of pH of the body. The symptoms of the disease appeared after 2 to 5 days to the exposure of bacterial strain and the duration of the disease is a few days [6].

DIAGNOSIS

Different tests are used for the diagnosis of cholera; cholera is diagnosed by a stool test by collecting the fecal sample of cholera patients. The colour and quality of the fecal sample of the patient help to diagnose cholera by visual testing. Malabsorption of fats in the feces and pH of the fecal sample used to diagnose cholera by different chemical tests. Microbiological tests are also used for diagnosis.

Dipstick Test for Diagnosis of Cholera

To diagnose cholera a crystal VC dipstick test is performed. In this test, the fresh sample of faces of the cholera patients is collected and two drops of the stool sample which is in liquid form supplemented in the vial and mixed well then few drops of the sample which is processed mixed and added in the test tube. Then the strip which is crystal VC dipped into the sample in the test tube and then the test results were analyzed [7].

Cholkit Test

In this test stool sample is used in liquid form, 5 drops of a stool sample were mixed with Tris- sodium chloride-tween and the ratio of both the samples 1:1 and mixed well both of these samples in a microcentrifuge and a cholkit is dipped in the tube for 15 minutes and on the kit, a control line and test line appeared simultaneously in red after test which shows positive results for *Vibrio cholerae* strain O1 and just one line appeared like a control line this means the negative results for the *V. cholerae* strain O1 [7].

Slide Agglutination Test

In this test a monoclonal antibody which is ICL-33 used for the detection of O1 strain of *Vibrio cholera* by the use of an agglutination slide TTGA to grow the different strains of *V. cholera* and the different strains of bacteria of *V. cholera* were cultured on the TTGA media plate at the room temperature of 37 ° C overnight. Then from this plate, a single colony of bacterial strain is picked and added on another glass slide with monoclonal antibody ICL-33 to carry out agglutination, if agglutination appears after two minutes this shows the positive results for *V. cholerea* strain [7].

Polymerase Chain Reaction

The toxin of the cholera is detected by Bead-Immunosorbent assay and PCR is used for the detection of the cholera toxin gene. The strain of *V. cholera* 01 is collected by culturing the samples of the patients and positive results were obtained by PCR. So PCR provides good and specific results for the diagnosis of cholera [8].

MANAGEMENT OF CHOLERA

Different vaccines, antibiotics, and different strategies are used for the management of cholera.

Vaccines

Cholera is the major problem causing diarrhea worldwide and different vaccines are used to control cholera.

Killed Oral Cholera Vaccine

There are some OCV that was approved by the World Health Organization and different vaccines have different efficiency to control the cholera disease. Some OCVs include Dukoral, Shanchol, and Euvichol, mORC-Vax, and Oravacs. These vaccines are used in different countries. Different doses administered at different ages of all vaccines [9]

Dukoral

This Dukoral vaccine is administered with a buffer which is sodium hydrogen carbonate solution and before and after the administration of vaccine food and drink is avoided. At the age of more than six 2 doses of the vaccine are given to the patient after two weeks, if the patient is 2-6 years old then the dose of vaccine is given after 6 months [10].

Shanchol

This vaccine is administered without any oral buffer and after two years dosses are given to the patient and at the age of 1 year after 14 days the dose of vaccine is given to the patient.

Euvichol

For this vaccine, no oral buffer required, and at the age of 1 year after 14 days dose of vaccine is repeated.

Rotavirus Vaccine

This vaccine is injected at an early age before 7-8 years to control the diarrhoea.

Oral Rehydration Therapy

This therapy is highly effective. In this rice-based therapy, solutions are used and the most used solution is Ringer's lactate and this solution is used with Potassium [11].

Antibiotics

Different antibiotics are used to prevent cholera, which includes Tetracycline, erythromycin, Chloramphenicol, and ciprofloxacin, A few of these antibiotics show good results and few may not.

PREVENTIONS

Some preventive measures are taken to reduce the cholera disease which includes the use of hygienic water, hygienic food, boiled and filtered water, and good sanitation.

CONSENT FOR PUBLICATION

Not applicable.

CONFLICT OF INTEREST

The authors declare no conflict of interest, financial or otherwise.

ACKNOWLEDGEMENTS

Declared none.

REFERENCES

[1]   Phelps M, Perner ML, Pitzer VE, Andreasen V, Jensen PKM, Simonsen L. Cholera epidemics of the past offer new insights into an old enemy. J Infect Dis 2018; 217(4): 641-9.
[http://dx.doi.org/10.1093/infdis/jix602] [PMID: 29165706]

[2]   Maina AN, Mwaura FB, Oyugi J, Goulding D, Toribio AL, Kariuki S. Characterization of *Vibrio cholerae* bacteriophages isolated from the environmental waters of the Lake Victoria region of Kenya. Curr Microbiol 2014; 68(1): 64-70.
[http://dx.doi.org/10.1007/s00284-013-0447-x] [PMID: 23982202]

[3]   Chowdhury F, Mather AE, Begum YA, *et al. Vibrio cholerae* serogroup O139: isolation from cholera patients and asymptomatic household family members in Bangladesh between 2013 and 2014. PLoS Negl Trop Dis 2015; 9(11)e0004183
[http://dx.doi.org/10.1371/journal.pntd.0004183] [PMID: 26562418]

[4]   Albert MJ, Ansaruzzaman M, Bardhan PK, Faruque A, Faruque SM, Islam M, *et al.* Large epidemic of cholera-like disease in Bangladesh caused by *Vibrio cholerae* 0139 synonym Bengal. Lancet 1993; 342(8868): 387-90.
[http://dx.doi.org/10.1016/0140-6736(93)92811-7] [PMID: 8101899]

[5]   Chiappelli F, Khakshooy A, Balenton N. Clinical Immunology of Cholera - Current Trends and Directions for Future Advancement. Bioinformation 2017; 13(10): 352-5.
[http://dx.doi.org/10.6026/97320630013352] [PMID: 29162969]

[6]   Lucien MAB, Schaad N, Steenland MW, *et al.* Identifying the most sensitive and specific sign and symptom combinations for cholera: results from an analysis of laboratory-based surveillance data from Haiti, 2012-2013. Am J Trop Med Hyg 2015; 92(4): 758-64.
[http://dx.doi.org/10.4269/ajtmh.14-0429] [PMID: 25732682]

[7]   Sayeed M, Islam K, Hossain M, Akter N, Alam M, Sultana N, *et al.* 2018.

[8]   Greig DR, Hickey TJ, Boxall MD, *et al.* A real-time multiplex PCR for the identification and typing of *Vibrio cholerae.* Diagn Microbiol Infect Dis 2018; 90(3): 171-6.
[http://dx.doi.org/10.1016/j.diagmicrobio.2017.11.017] [PMID: 29274667]

[9]   Peak CM, Reilly AL, Azman AS, Buckee CO. Prolonging herd immunity to cholera *via* vaccination: Accounting for human mobility and waning vaccine effects. PLoS Negl Trop Dis 2018; 12(2)e0006257
[http://dx.doi.org/10.1371/journal.pntd.0006257] [PMID: 29489815]

[10]   van Splunter M, van Hoffen E, Floris-Vollenbroek EG, *et al.* Oral cholera vaccination promotes homing of IgA$^+$ memory B cells to the large intestine and the respiratory tract. Mucosal Immunol 2018; 11(4): 1254-64.
[http://dx.doi.org/10.1038/s41385-018-0006-7] [PMID: 29467446]

[11]   Gore SM, Fontaine O, Pierce NF. Impact of rice based oral rehydration solution on stool output and duration of diarrhoea: meta-analysis of 13 clinical trials. BMJ 1992; 304(6822): 287-91.
[http://dx.doi.org/10.1136/bmj.304.6822.287] [PMID: 1531430]

CHAPTER 29

Impetigo: A Skin Infection Caused by *Streptococci* and *Staphylococci*

Muhammad Imran Qadir[*] and **Iqra Jamshaid**

Institute of Molecular Biology & Biotechnology, Bahauddin Zakariya University, Multan, Pakistan

Abstract: Impetigo is a skin infection which is caused by a bacterial strain of *Streptococcus* and *Staphylococcus*. Impetigo has two types, bullous impetigo, and non-bullous impetigo. Impetigo is more common in children however it can affect any age. It begins with a small pimple and ends with blisters which break the skin and thus cause infection. Treatment of impetigo includes topical antibiotics in which fusidic acid and mupirocin have used cream and can be applied on site of infection. Oral antibiotics include erythromycin, penicillin, and flucloxacillin. But the oral antibiotics are not as effective as topical antibiotics. But when the topical antibiotics show no results then oral antibiotic is used.

Keywords: Diagnosis, Impetigo, Treatment, Types.

INTRODUCTION

Impetigo is a bacterial skin infection which is due to two strains of bacteria named *Streptococcus* and *Staphylococcus*. These two bacteria release a toxin that breakdown the skin forming pustules. This disease is more common in children than in adults. These are two forms of impetigo non-bullous impetigo, bullous impetigo [1].

PREVALENCE

Impetigo is usually spread by direct contact. In the United Kingdom, the annual spreading of impetigo was 2.8% in the children at the age of 4 years and 1.6% at the age of 5 to 15 years. Almost 70% of cases were nonbullous impetigo and patients transmitted this disease further to themselves and others by damage an infected area [2]. Thus the infection is spread mostly through schools and daycare

[*] **Corresponding author Muhammad Imran Qadir:** Institute of Molecular Biology and Biotechnology, Bahauddin Zakariya University, Multan, Pakistan; Tel: +92-61-9210071; Ext. 1920; Fax: +92-61-9210068; E-mail: mrimranqadir@hotmail.com

Muhammad Imran Qadir (Ed.)
All rights reserved-© 2020 Bentham Science Publishers

centers. The infection is occurring mostly in poor hygiene, crowded environment, and mostly in summer [3].

DIAGNOSIS

Non-bullous Impetigo

It is due to *Streptococcus pyogenes* or by both staph and strep .5-10% is usually due to strap bacteria alone. Red spots are formed on the skin around nose and mouth and in this way small pustules are formed which in the form of clusters spread on the other area of skin then this pustule rapture and formed a yellow crust on the skin they are not painful but fretful. When they recover they look like a red spot they leave a trauma on the skin. It is usually in the age of 2 years children [4].

Ecthyma

It is due to either *Streptococcus pyogenes* or *Staphylococcus aureus* or both types of bacteria. In this small pus-filled sores are formed which have a thicker crust, it is more severe than the other type of impetigo because the sore can go deep into the skin. The sore becomes large and deep and thus formed a reddish-purple skin at the site of infection. Mostly occur around buttocks, thighs, legs, ankles, and feet. If non-bullous and bullous impetigo leaves untreated they formed ecthyma which recovers slowly and thus left a trauma on the skin [5].

Bullous Impetigo

It is due to *S. aureus* bacteria which form larger pustules that further form a bullae and this bullae is filled with fluid. When they split yellow crust with ejaculation results. It mostly occurs around moist areas, for example, diaper area, axillae, and neck fold. Symptoms may include fever, weakness, and diarrhea [6].

TREATMENT

The basic aim of treatment includes preventing the further transmission of infection within the patients and others. Treatment should have limited side effects, inexpensive and effective. Topical antibodies have advantages over the oral antibiotic but some patients are more susceptible to these antibodies [7].

TOPICAL ANTIBIOTICS

For the treatment of impetigo, three studies concluded that topical antibodies are more effective than oral antibiotics because they can apply on skin anywhere and do not cause any adverse effects. Mupirocin and fusidic acid are effective and well-tolerated against them. Adverse effects of topical antibodies were uncommon and mild when present [8].

Fusidic Acid

It is more effective against the strains of *S. aureus* bacteria because it penetrates the skin. It is less effective against Streptococcus. Gram-negative bacteria have resistance to fusidic acid. It is a steroid antibiotic often given in forms of cream, tablets, eye drops, or injections [9].

Mupirocin

It is topical antibiotics and used as a cream. It is effective against *S. aureus* and also effective against methicillin which causes impetigo or folliculitis. It contains benzyl alcohol, cetyl alcohol, and stearyl alcohol. The patients who are sensitive to these ambient are recommended to use emollient. Both fusidic acid and mupirocin are effective as compared to oral antibiotics [10].

ORAL ANTIBIOTICS

When topical antibodies do not show results then oral antibodies are used. For example, erythromycin, penicillin, and flucloxacillin. These antibiotics are used in the past but due to their replacement with drug resistance, they are not used routinely. Resistance rates vary regionally so it is recommended to check the resistance pattern of appropriate antibiotics [7].

CONSENT FOR PUBLICATION

Not applicable.

CONFLICT OF INTEREST

The authors declare no conflict of interest, financial or otherwise.

ACKNOWLEDGEMENTS

Declared none.

REFERENCES

[1]   Pereira LB. Impetigo - review. An Bras Dermatol 2014; 89(2): 293-9.
       [http://dx.doi.org/10.1590/abd1806-4841.20142283] [PMID: 24770507]

[2]   Romani L, Steer AC, Whitfeld MJ, Kaldor JM. Prevalence of scabies and impetigo worldwide: a systematic review. Lancet Infect Dis 2015; 15(8): 960-7.
[http://dx.doi.org/10.1016/S1473-3099(15)00132-2] [PMID: 26088526]

[3]   Brown J, Shriner DL, Schwartz RA, Janniger CK. Impetigo: an update. Int J Dermatol 2003; 42(4): 251-5.
[http://dx.doi.org/10.1046/j.1365-4362.2003.01647.x] [PMID: 12694487]

[4]   Verduin C, van Suijlekom-Smit LW, van der Wouden JC, Leeuwen HV, Nouwen J, Op M, *et al.* Severity of Nonbullous.

[5]   Nolting S, Strauss WB. Treatment of impetigo and ecthyma. A comparison of sulconazole with miconazole. Int J Dermatol 1988; 27(10): 716-9.
[http://dx.doi.org/10.1111/j.1365-4362.1988.tb01273.x] [PMID: 3069760]

[6]   Stanley JR, Amagai M. Pemphigus, bullous impetigo, and the staphylococcal scalded-skin syndrome. N Engl J Med 2006; 355(17): 1800-10.
[http://dx.doi.org/10.1056/NEJMra061111] [PMID: 17065642]

[7]   Carruthers R. Prescribing antibiotics for impetigo. Drugs 1988; 36(3): 364-9.
[http://dx.doi.org/10.2165/00003495-198836030-00006] [PMID: 3056694]

[8]   Burnett JW. The route of antibiotic administration in superficial impetigo. N Engl J Med 1963; 268(2): 72-5.
[http://dx.doi.org/10.1056/NEJM196301102680203] [PMID: 14017141]

[9]   Cole C, Gazewood J. Diagnosis and treatment of impetigo. Am Fam Physician 2007; 75(6): 859-64.
[PMID: 17390597]

[10]   Hartman-Adams H, Banvard C, Juckett G. Impetigo: diagnosis and treatment. Am Fam Physician 2014; 90(4): 229-35.
[PMID: 25250996]

CHAPTER 30

Lyme Disease: A *Borrelia Burgdorferi* Infection

Muhammad Imran Qadir[*] and **Sidra Noureen**

Institute of Molecular Biology & Biotechnology, Bahauddin Zakariya University, Multan, Pakistan

Abstract: Lyme disease is an infection that is caused by ticks and strains of bacteria *Borrelia burgdorferi*. The disease is transmitted to humans and also to the livestock and pets through ticks. Symptoms of this disease are headache, fever, and other skin infections. Diagnosis of this disease is difficult but can be diagnosed by ELISA and western blot tests. Different types of antibiotics are used for the treatment of Lyme disease. Through drugs and antibiotics, recovery begins sooner.

Keywords: Causes, Lyme disease, Symptoms, Treatment.

INTRODUCTION

Lyme disease is the infection that is caused by the bite of the deer tick. Several strains of bacteria also cause this disease. The main cause of this disease is *Borrelia burgdorferi*. Lyme disease was first discovered and recognized in 1874 and it occurs mostly in the children. It is the vector-borne disease and most common in the US. It is transmitted to humans when the ticks bite them. It is transmitted only when the ticks came in contact with humans. It is not transmitted from person to person. Multiple organs are disturbed due to this infection [1]. The disease is rare but fatal.

SYMPTOMS

Erythema Migrans

It is the first symptom of the disease. The skin becomes red or red rash appears on the area where tick bites. The rash area became more highlighted with time if not treated with antibiotics. The most common symptoms accompanied headache, fever, fatigue [2].

---

[*] **Corresponding author Muhammad Imran Qadir:** Institute of Molecular Biology and Biotechnology, Bahauddin Zakariya University, Multan, Pakistan; Tel: +92-61-9210071; Ext. 1920; Fax: +92-61-9210068; E-mail: mrimranqadir@hotmail.com

Muhammad Imran Qadir (Ed.)
All rights reserved-© 2020 Bentham Science Publishers

Arthritis

If the disease left untreated after the bite of a tick, the infection may spread to joints. The joints became swollen and more painful and this pain lasts for weeks or even months.

Heart Problem

Irregular heartbeat and dizziness occur if the disease is not treated.

Neurological and Other Symptoms

The symptoms are changes in sleeping habits, fatigue. Other symptoms are the inflammation of eyes and joints pain and hepatitis.

DIAGNOSIS

Its diagnosis is difficult sometimes. Doctors may ask for genetic reports. Lab test identifies bacteria responsible for the disease. Ticks are important clues for diagnosis [3].

They test includes:

- ELISA detects antibodies. Sometimes, false-positive results occur.
- Western blot testing is also helpful. A positive test confirms the diagnosis [4].

TREATMENT

For treatment, antibiotics are used:

- Intravenous antibiotics are used but they can cause side effects leading to diarrhea [5]. When few doses of these antibiotics are given, the disease is recovered but it may still have many symptoms.
- The FDA warns against the use of bismacine. Bismacine, also known as chromacine, shave bismuth-containing its toxic level. Bismacine can cause bismuth poisoning, which may lead to heart and kidney failure.
- Oral antibiotics are also used.

CONSENT FOR PUBLICATION

Not applicable.

CONFLICT OF INTEREST

The authors declare no conflict of interest, financial or otherwise.

ACKNOWLEDGEMENTS

Declared none.

REFERENCES

[1]   Marzec NS, Nelson C, Waldron PR, *et al.* Serious Bacterial Infections Acquired During Treatment of Patients Given a Diagnosis of Chronic Lyme Disease - United States. MMWR Morb Mortal Wkly Rep 2017; 66(23): 607-9.
[http://dx.doi.org/10.15585/mmwr.mm6623a3] [PMID: 28617768]

[2]   Doshi S, Keilp JG, Strobino B, McElhiney M, Rabkin J, Fallon BA. Depressive symptoms and suicidal ideation among symptomatic patients with a history of Lyme disease *versus* two comparison groups. Psychosomatics 2018; 59(5): 481-9.
[http://dx.doi.org/10.1016/j.psym.2018.02.004] [PMID: 29606281]

[3]   Branda JA, Strle K, Nigrovic LE, *et al.* Evaluation of modified 2-tiered serodiagnostic testing algorithms for early Lyme disease. Clin Infect Dis 2017; 64(8): 1074-80.
[http://dx.doi.org/10.1093/cid/cix043] [PMID: 28329259]

[4]   Miller GL, Craven RB, Bailey RE, Tsai TF. The epidemiology of Lyme disease in the United States 1987-1988. Lab Med 2016; 21(5): 285-9.
[http://dx.doi.org/10.1093/labmed/21.5.285]

[5]   Pavia CS, Plummer MM. Was it authentic Lyme disease or some other disorder? Pathog Dis 2017; 75(3)
[http://dx.doi.org/10.1093/femspd/ftx028] [PMID: 28369369]

CHAPTER 31

Peptic Ulcer: A *Helicobacter Pylori* Infection

Muhammad Imran Qadir[*] and **Fatima Rehan**

Institute of Molecular Biology & Biotechnology, Bahauddin Zakariya University, Multan, Pakistan

Abstract: *Helicobacter pylori* infection which is a constantly occurring disease causes damage to normal regulation and function of gastric acid. It was estimated that peptic ulcer infection was developed in about only 15% of persons that were infected with *Helicobacter pylori*. Burning, epigastric pain, and nocturnal pain after food intake are typical symptoms. Urea breath test, stool antigen test, or an endoscopic biopsy and ELISA may be performed as a diagnostic test for confirmation of occurrence of *Helicobacter pylori infection* in peptic ulcer patients. Management for peptic ulcer infection includes drug treatment and surgery.

Keywords: Diagnosis Test, *H. pylori*, Managements, Peptic Ulcer.

INTRODUCTION

Peptic ulcer infection occurs in the gastrointestinal tract that initially damages mucus secretion, then damages pepsin and gastric enzyme secretion. In the stomach and duodenum, it is commonly present and it is less commonly occurs in the lower esophagus. Gastric acid secretion initiates the process of digestion in the body and plays a unique role as the first line of defense against many microorganisms such as food-borne microbes. *Helicobacter pylori* infection which is a constantly occurring disease causes damage to normal regulation and function of gastric acid. The successful culture of *Campylobacter pylori* was first examined with its taxonomic features in detail. Due to minor differences in features with other campylobacter and its exceptional features, *C. pylori* was named *Helicobacter pylori*. The person with peptic ulcer harbors the organism only in gastric epithelium. *H. pylori* cluster around cells and are not found in the blood. In the study, it was concluded that there is a high risk of gastric cancer for patients with gastric ulcers infected by *Helicobacter pylori* [1].

[*] **Corresponding author Muhammad Imran Qadir:** Institute of Molecular Biology and Biotechnology, Bahauddin Zakariya University, Multan, Pakistan; Tel: +92-61-9210071; Ext. 1920; Fax: +92-61-9210068; E-mail: mrimranqadir@hotmail.com

Muhammad Imran Qadir (Ed.)
All rights reserved-© 2020 Bentham Science Publishers

PREVALENCE AND CAUSES

The major cause of peptic ulcers includes *H. pylori* infection and the other one is non-steroidal anti-inflammatory drugs (NSAIDs). It was estimated that peptic ulcer infection was developed in about only 10 to 15 percent of people that were infected due to *H. pylori*. Elimination of residing *H. pylori* lowers the risk of ulcer formation from fifty-nine to four percent in patients with peptic ulcer. Peptic ulcer infection occurs at the age between 25 and 64 years in 70 percent of patients. The estimation of annual health care cost of the disease is about $ 10 billion in the United States but through maximum use of proton pump inhibitors minimizes the rate of *H. pylori* infection directly or indirectly. Hepatic cirrhosis, tuberculosis, chronic renal failure, Crohn's disease, sarcoidosis, cytomegalovirus, and myeloproliferative disorder are risk factors associated with peptic ulcer disease [2].

SYMPTOMS

Specific findings for peptic ulcer helpful in the diagnosis are ITS distinctive symptoms of peptic ulcer disease include burning epigastric pain; pain occurring on an empty stomach or two to five hours after meals; and nocturnal pain after food intake. Less common features observed as peptic ulcer symptoms include vomiting, intolerance of fatty foods, heartburn, indigestion, loss of appetite, and positive family history. The physical diagnosis is also helpful to reduce the possibility of the occurrence of ulcers.

Symptoms of peptic ulcer infection vary among individual populations. Abdominal pain is absent in older patients with peptic ulcers. Fear of food intake leads to weight loss is characteristic of gastric ulcers [3].

DIAGNOSIS

For the diagnosis of peptic ulcer, proper physical examination of the patient is required to perform. The person with age younger than 55 years comes under less risk level of peptic infection. Recommended tests for peptic ulcer disease should be based on symptoms of patients. Enzyme-linked immunosorbent assay (ELISA), urea breath test, stool antigen test, or an endoscopic biopsy performed as a diagnostic test for confirmation of the presence of *H. pylori* in peptic ulcer patient.

ELISA is useful for initial infection diagnosis and diagnosis in large population surveys. The stool antigen test is highly accurate in specificity and sensitivity like the urea breath test. However, the urea breath test is not cheaper and convenient in equipment like the stool antigen test. Though, both tests performed to confirm suppression of *H. pylori.* Endoscopy is preferred if a patient of 55 years or more showing continuous symptoms of peptic ulcer infection. The therapy eradicates the ulcer formation within one or two weeks of endoscopy [4].

MANAGEMENT

Management for peptic ulcer infection includes treatment and surgery. Eradication of *Helicobacter pylori*, histamine H2 blockers, proton pump inhibitors is used as a treatment for the management of peptic ulcer disease. Eradication therapy is recommended for about 10 to 14 days and 1, 5, and 7 days for short duration treatment. The rate of eradication is eighty to ninety percent or more. Histamine H2 blockers are administrated for duodenal ulcers and after four weeks, the healing rate is 70 to 80 percent and 87 to 94 percent healing after eight weeks of administration. Treatment duration of proton pump inhibitor for duodenal ulcer is 4 weeks and the healing rate is 80 to 100 percent.

Surgery is recommended for the patient who had multiple medications. The patients who are not affecting with medication with no response and those at complications with high risk are also recommended for surgery. Surgery for duodenal ulcers includes highly selective vagotomy, truncal vagotomy, partial gastrectomy, and selective vagotomy. Partial gastrectomy with gastroduodenal anastomosis is recommended for gastric ulcers [5].

CONSENT FOR PUBLICATION

Not applicable.

CONFLICT OF INTEREST

The authors declare no conflict of interest, financial or otherwise.

ACKNOWLEDGEMENTS

Declared none.

REFERENCES

[1]   Peterson WL. *Helicobacter pylori* and peptic ulcer disease. N Engl J Med 1991; 324(15): 1043-8.
        [http://dx.doi.org/10.1056/NEJM199104113241507] [PMID: 2005942]

[2]   Ziegler AB. The role of proton pump inhibitors in acute stress ulcer prophylaxis in mechanically ventilated patients. Dimens Crit Care Nurs 2005; 24(3): 109-14.
        [http://dx.doi.org/10.1097/00003465-200505000-00001] [PMID: 15912057]

[3]   Ramakrishnan K, Salinas RC. Peptic ulcer disease. Am Fam Physician 2007; 76(7): 1005-12.
        [PMID: 17956071]

[4]   Fashner J, Gitu AC. Diagnosis and Treatment of Peptic Ulcer Disease and H. pylori Infection. Am Fam Physician 2015; 91(4): 236-42.

[PMID: 25955624]

[5]   Behrman SW. Management of complicated peptic ulcer disease. Arch Surg 2005; 140(2): 201-8.
[http://dx.doi.org/10.1001/archsurg.140.2.201] [PMID: 15724004]

CHAPTER 32

Toxic Shock Syndrome: A Condition Caused by Endotoxin Produced by *Staphylococcus Aureus*

Muhammad Imran Qadir[*] and **Aleena Ahmad Somroo**

Institute of Molecular Biology & Biotechnology, Bahauddin Zakariya University, Multan, Pakistan

Abstract: Toxic shock syndrome is an uncommon but life-threatening disease which is caused by the poisonous endotoxin (TSS-1) produced by *Staphylococcus aureus* bacteria. Toxic shock syndrome was first described in children in the 1976. This disease is more common in women than in men. Infection is caused due to the entrance of bacteria in the body through skin opening such as cuts or wounds or due to poorly conducted skin surgery, skin-burn, and skin infection. Prevalence of *S.aureus* colonization and antibodies by age, geographical area there was no significant difference found in the rate of toxigenicity and colonization while the population study prevalence was found to be 26%. Symptoms of TSS were skin rashes, headache, fever, vomiting, diarrhea, including neurological disturbance and the central nervous system disturbance along with organ failure. The diagnosis was done using Cole and Shakespeare's criteria proposed for toxic shock syndrome it can be also diagnosis from body fluids test and urine test. Management includes seven R's which are very important for managing the toxic shock syndrome.

Keywords: Cole and Shakespeare, Endotoxin, Management, Shock, Skin-Burn, "*Staphylococcus aureus*", Toxigenicity, Toxin, TSS-1.

INTRODUCTION

Toxic shock syndrome is a life-threatening disease that is caused due to the toxins produced in response to group A *Staphylococcus* infection or *staphylococcus aureus*. It is also known as *Staphylococcus* pyogenes. It is further characterized by fever, skin rash, hypotension, and failure of more than one organ after acute "illness" including diarrhea, vomiting. The toxic syndrome was first described in children in the late 19th century *i.e.* 1976. This disease is commonly found in women [1].

[*] **Corresponding author Muhammad Imran Qadir:** Institute of Molecular Biology and Biotechnology, Bahauddin Zakariya University, Multan, Pakistan; Tel: +92-61-9210071; Ext. 1920; Fax: +92-61-9210068; E-mail: mrimranqadir@hotmail.com

Muhammad Imran Qadir (Ed.)
All rights reserved-© 2020 Bentham Science Publishers

Infection is caused when bacteria enter into the body through open skin such as sore, cuts, or any other wounds. Risk factors for becoming susceptible to this disease are skin infection, burn, or surgery [2].

Prevalence of *S. aureus* colonization and antibodies by geographical location, age, there were no significant differences found in the rate of colony-forming and toxigenicity according to the geographical area that was found, while the prevalence for a population study was found to be 26% of subjects [3].

SYMPTOMS

Toxic shock syndrome shows a variety of symptoms which are followed by vomiting, diarrhea, hypotension, and cold sweats, dizziness, unconscious, and later is continued by the clinical manifestation of staphylococcal TSS, myalgia, high fever and skin, and the mucous membrane is involved early. Rashes appear on the skin which resembles suntan like appearances. After a few days "desquamation" occurs on the face, palm, and extreme areas. Mucous involvement occurs as a sore throat and a strawberry tongue. Gastrointestinal abnormalities may also develop in early illness. Cardiac and renal abnormalities can be also found in this disease [4].

DIAGNOSIS

Studies conducted by [5] in which 13 children were selected and their conditions were examined, it was concluded that all children were presented with the signs of pyrexia and septic shock and rash appeared in 11 out of 13 youngsters and 85% shows the signs of central nervous system disturbance such as drowsiness and unconsciousness on further investigation 10 children were hyponatremic and 9 were lymphopaenic at the time of diagnosis. The diagnosis was done using Cole and Shakespeare's criteria for TSS.

MANAGEMENT

The management of toxic shock syndrome includes seven R's of management which are recognition which is followed by resuscitation, removal of the source of infection, rational choice of antibiotics, the role of adjuvant management: including clindamycin, intervenous immunoglobin, review progress and the reduction of risk of secondary cases in close contacts [6]. Currently, the research done for the therapy of the "toxic shock syndrome" monoclonal antibodies are developed which can neutralize the TSST-1 and the other antigen produced, the use of ligands TLR2 and fixed antibodies which have high affinity to extract the endotoxin are being directed.

CONSENT FOR PUBLICATION

Not applicable.

CONFLICT OF INTEREST

The authors declare no conflict of interest, financial or otherwise.

ACKNOWLEDGEMENTS

Declared none.

REFERENCES

[1]   Venkataraman R. Toxic Shock Syndrome Background, Pathophysiology, Etiology.pdf. [updated 13/03/17; cited 2018 26 march]; Available from: https://emedicine.medscape.com/article/169177-overview

[2]   Higuera V. Toxic shock syndrome: symptoms, diagnosis, and treatment pdf 2016. https://www.healthline.com/health/toxic-shock-syndrome

[3]   Parsonnet J, Hansmann MA, Delaney ML, *et al.* Prevalence of toxic shock syndrome toxin 1-producing *Staphylococcus aureus* and the presence of antibodies to this superantigen in menstruating women. J Clin Microbiol 2005; 43(9): 4628-34.
[http://dx.doi.org/10.1128/JCM.43.9.4628-4634.2005] [PMID: 16145118]

[4]   Reiss MA. Toxic shock syndrome. Prim Care Update Ob Gyns 2000; 7(3): 85-90.
[http://dx.doi.org/10.1016/S1068-607X(00)00027-5] [PMID: 10840210]

[5]   White MC, Thornton K, Young AE. Early diagnosis and treatment of toxic shock syndrome in paediatric burns. Burns 2005; 31(2): 193-7.
[http://dx.doi.org/10.1016/j.burns.2004.09.017] [PMID: 15683692]

[6]   Wilkins AL, Steer AC, Smeesters PR, Curtis N. Toxic shock syndrome - the seven Rs of management and treatment. J Infect 2017; 74 (Suppl. 1): S147-52.
[http://dx.doi.org/10.1016/S0163-4453(17)30206-2] [PMID: 28646955]

CHAPTER 33

Scarlet Fever: An Infection Symptomized by Red Rash All Over the Body with High Fever

Muhammad Imran Qadir[*] and **Iqra Ali Yameen**

Institute of Molecular Biology & Biotechnology, Bahauddin Zakariya University, Multan, Pakistan

Abstract: Scarlet fever is a bacterial disease caused by the *streptococcus* family. *streptococcus* pyogenes is an infectious agent in this disease. This bacteria produces streptococcal pyrogenic endotoxins SPEs that causes a red rash and high fever. Common symptoms seen in patients suffering from scarlet fever are swollen tonsils, high fever, red folding in arms, and elbows. Scarlet fever mostly occurs in children and sometimes it also affects adults. In past decades, the mortality rate due to scarlet fever was 10-25 percent but now it is reduced to 1% due to antibiotics. Diagnosis against scarlet fever is done by different methods like throat swab specimen detection and antigen screening method. For the treatment of scarlet fever, no vaccines are present. Antibiotics and hygienic lifestyle are recommended to lower the severity of scarlet fever.

Keywords: Antibiotics, Endotoxins, High Fever, Scarlet Fever, *streptococcus* pyogenes.

INTRODUCTION

Scarlatina or scarlet fever is an infectious disease that causes a red rash all over the body with a high fever. Scarlet fever is caused by the group A *streptococcus* (GAS) bacteria that is present in our nasal cavity and throat. The same bacterial strains of GAS also causes strep throat disease in individuals. The group A *streptococcus* bacteria includes several bacterial strains but *streptococcus* pyogenes is more dangerous besides all others. This is a *Gram*+ve bacteria that produce streptococcal pyrogenic exotoxins SPEs. This endotoxin causes a red rash all over the body, strawberry-like tongue appearance with swollen papillae, red rash folding at the elbow, and pits is a sign of scarlet fever [1]. Common symptoms seen after 1 to 4 days in scarlet fever includes flushed face, strawberry tongue, fever above 101^0F, swollen tonsils, red lines around the elbow, swollen

[*] **Corresponding author Muhammad Imran Qadir:** Institute of Molecular Biology and Biotechnology, Bahauddin Zakariya University, Multan, Pakistan; Tel: +92-61-9210071; Ext. 1920; Fax: +92-61-9210068; E-mail: mrimranqadir@hotmail.com

Muhammad Imran Qadir (Ed.)
All rights reserved-© 2020 Bentham Science Publishers

lymph nodes, chill, headache followed by nausea. The rash starts from the stomach and chest then spreads all over the body. This lasts for 2 - 7 days if complete treatment is used [2]. *streptococcus* pyogenes also give rise to several diseases like tonsils, pharyngitis, toxic shock, and rheumatic fever and heart diseases. It mainly affects children between the ages of 5 to 10 years. Scarlet fever was a common disease in recent past years. It is a toxin-mediated disease that has been deadly affecting the entire world. Scarlet fever disease was pandemic in Asia. The incidence rate of scarlet fever has been increasing in different countries due to the resistance of infectious agents against antibiotics. In South Korean from 2008 to 2015 disease rate suddenly increased from 0.3 to 13.7 cases per 10,0000 [3]. It was reported that a higher disease rate in South Korea is due to resistance against tetracycline antibiotics. Scarlet fever was first reported in Scotland and England in 1661. Genomic analysis was performed to check the statics of scarlet fever in correspondence to invasive diseases of the Group A streptococcal strains [4]. The worldwide occurrence of scarlet fever within the past 20 years has declined due to the emergence of new generations of antibiotics and medicine with a high spectrum range against group A *streptococcus* bacterial strains. The occurrence of scarlet fever depends upon the *emm* type that is an adhesion fimbriae protein transcribed by special gene sequences. Higher genetic variations in *emm* make it resistant towards a class of antibiotics. Different *emm* types dominate in different parts of the world. Scarlet fever 12 clones of *emm* especially ICE_*emm* 12 that is tetracycline resistance and ICE_HKU 397 are commonly present two elements of emm12 in China. It was the common disease of childhood in past decades that also affects adults. Now a day's recent advancement in antibiotics has made it less dangerous. Up till now only compromised antibiotics are used for scarlet fever, no vaccines are available against this disease.

CAUSES AND SYMPTOMS

Scarlet fever is caused by group A *streptococcus* (GAS) bacteria. Among these GAS bacteria, *streptococcus* pyogenes are most common that produce all signs of scarlet fever especially rashes and high fever. *streptococcus* pyogenes bacteria produces "streptococcal pyrogenic endotoxins" (SPEs) that circulate with bloodstreams and causes flushed cheeks with pale lips, rash on chest and trunk, swollen tonsils and fever above 100 ^{0}F. Proteins produced by *streptococcus* pyogenes were first termed as erythrogenic toxins but nowadays more accurately known as pyrogenic endotoxins. Each bacterial strain produces more than 2 to 3 different types of endotoxins. Eleven such endotoxins have been identified in different case studies, while in scarlet fever, a mixture of endotoxin SpeA, streptococcal pyrogenic endotoxin C and SSA are mostly present. These SPEs are seen to play a role in toxic shock syndrome, rheumatic fever, and pharyngitis [5].

DIAGNOSIS

Diagnosis of scarlet fever depends upon scoring system that is designed to enhance accuracy in the identification of *streptococcus* pyogenes and SPEs. Scoring depends upon the occurrence or absence of fever, rashes, swollen tonsils, and lymph nodes. The best scoring also involves patients' age and previous medical records. A golden method for diagnosis of scarlet fever is "throat swab specimen". Rapid antigen detection test and throat culture are commonly used now a day to evaluate the presence of an infectious agent that causes this disease. The first one is highly specific but it is not completely sensitive for the infectious agent and provides false-negative results. The golden standard that provides accurate results in the diagnosis of scarlet fever, is the throat swab culture. Other testing methods like serologic testing were also used for a short time but it does not provide clear results as the body takes approximately 2 to 3 weeks to develop antibodies against this infectious agent after the onset of infection [6].

MANAGEMENT

Scarlet fever is mostly treated as a self-limited illness, but the use of antibiotics lowers the severity and complexity of this disease by making a remarkable change in therapy. The use of antibiotic penicillin shortens the duration of fever up to one day, minimizes the chances of suffering from the worst condition of rheumatic fever [7]. The use of antibiotics prevents further complications of scarlet fever by reducing the chances of secondary infections. No vaccination is available against scarlet fever. Antibiotics like penicillin (oral), amoxicillin (oral), benzathine penicillin G (intramuscular), and for individuals with penicillin allergies cephalexin (oral) cephalosporin and cefadroxil are mostly recommended during this duration depending upon the condition of the patient. Penicillin due to its low cost, high efficiency, and best clinical guideline practices are commonly used that lowers the severity of fever and throat soreness.

CONSENT FOR PUBLICATION

Not applicable.

CONFLICT OF INTEREST

The authors declare no conflict of interest, financial or otherwise.

ACKNOWLEDGEMENTS

Declared none.

REFERENCES

[1]   Basetti S, Hodgson J, Rawson TM, Majeed A. Scarlet fever: a guide for general practitioners. London J Prim Care (Abingdon) 2017; 9(5): 77-9.
[http://dx.doi.org/10.1080/17571472.2017.1365677] [PMID: 29081840]

[2]   Campbell LR. Pharyngitis, Tonsillitis (Group A streptococcus), & Scarlet Fever A2 - Garfunkel, Lynn C.Pediatric Clinical Advisor. 2nd ed. Philadelphia: Mosby 2007; pp. 442-4.
[http://dx.doi.org/10.1016/B978-032303506-4.10253-6]

[3]   Duck-Woong P, Sun-Hee K, Jung-Wook P, Min-Ji K, Sun Ju C, Hye-Jung P, *et al.* Incidence and Characteristics of Scarlet Fever, South Korea, 2008–2015. *Emerging.* Infect Dis J 2017; 23: 658.

[4]   Chalker V, Jironkin A, Coelho J, *et al.* Genome analysis following a national increase in Scarlet Fever in England 2014. BMC Genomics 2017; 18(1): 224.
[http://dx.doi.org/10.1186/s12864-017-3603-z] [PMID: 28283023]

[5]   Quinn RW. Comprehensive review of morbidity and mortality trends for rheumatic fever, streptococcal disease, and scarlet fever: the decline of rheumatic fever. Rev Infect Dis 1989; 11(6): 928-53.
[http://dx.doi.org/10.1093/clinids/11.6.928] [PMID: 2690288]

[6]   Wessels MR. Pharyngitis and scarlet fever streptococcus pyogenes 2016; 1-10.

[7]   Shulman ST, Bisno AL, Clegg HW, *et al.* Clinical practice guideline for the diagnosis and management of group A *streptococcal pharyngitis*: 2012 update by the Infectious Diseases Society of America. Clin Infect Dis 2012; 55(10): e86-e102.
[http://dx.doi.org/10.1093/cid/cis629] [PMID: 22965026]

CHAPTER 34

Listeriosis: A Foodborne Disease Caused by *Listeria*

Muhammad Imran Qadir[*] and **Mahnoor Khan**

Institute of Molecular Biology & Biotechnology, Bahauddin Zakariya University, Multan, Pakistan

Abstract: Listeriosis is a foodborne disease. Bacteria of genus Listeria are responsible for this disease, especially *Listeria monocytogenes* which is a gram-positive bacterium and is active in the conditions needed to preserve food. The Mortality rate of listeriosis is 24%. Listeriosis is a serious threat to pregnant women and persons who are Immuno deficient. Symptoms of listeriosis are fever, flu, brain abscess, the tremor, Cranial nerve deficits, respiratory distress, jaundice, rash, or lethargy, *etc.* Diagnosis is done by culturing the organism from the blood and in the treatment, many antibiotics are given alone or sometimes in combination with two or more. Treatment of trimethoprim/sulfamethoxazole (TMP/SMX) is given as alternate to patients who have allergies with using penicillin.

Keywords: Antibiotics, Foodborne Disease, *Listeria monocytogenes*Listeriosis..

INTRODUCTION

Listeriosis is a food poisoning disease caused by bacterium *Listeria* that contaminates the food. Listeriosis is a human and animal disease. In humans, it is a foodborne disease. Pathogenic bacteria are responsible for this disease which belongs to the genus *Listeria.* Seven species of genus Listeria are found. And among seven species of this genus, only two are considered as the pathogenic [1]. Listeriosis is a serious threat, especially to immunodeficient persons. Almost 99% of cases of listeriosis in humans are caused by unhealthy and contaminated food [2]. In pregnancy, *Listeriosis* occurs at all stages [3].

Listeria monocytogenes is a gram-positive bacterium. It is an intracellular pathogen and is non-spore forming which is commonly found in our environment and a causative organism of many foodborne diseases. Listeria species can grow in vast range and their growing conditions, including the temperature between 1-

[*] **Corresponding author Muhammad Imran Qadir:** Institute of Molecular Biology and Biotechnology, Bahauddin Zakariya University, Multan, Pakistan, Tel. +92-61-9210071; Ext. 1920; Fax: +92-61-9210068; E-mail: mrimranqadir@hotmail.com

Muhammad Imran Qadir (Ed.)
All rights reserved-© 2020 Bentham Science Publishers

46 degrees Celsius, Salt concentrations up to 9-10%, and pH 4.3-9.6. These are the conditions that are used to preserve food and the bacteria are active and living in such conditions so it is a serious problem to the food. The mortality rate of listeriosis is 24%. Listeriosis is mostly found in pregnant women (in the fetus), also found in Immunodeficient persons, *Listeria* has an intracellular life cycle is intracellular, which makes it a unique pathogen. When we ingest contaminated food, *Listeria* is phagocytosed by the gastrointestinal cells and then it enters the host without upsetting the gastrointestinal tract [4]. When it reaches the cytoplasm of the host, it frequently divides and adjacent cells then may ingest it. *Listeria* can spread and multiply by these steps without exposing them to antibodies like neutrophils. That's why maternal *Listeria* can be of any sort like mild or dangerous. Cell-mediated immunity is the host's defense response against *Listeria* is the cell-mediated immunity, and many conditions reduce this immunity like pregnancy can cause early listerial infection [3].

SYMPTOMS

In many cases, mild maternal illness is reported and sometimes it can be severe. Some common symptoms of *Listeriosis* are:

Fever, 2nd most common symptom is Flu and white blood cells range from 3900 to 33,800cells/mm^3. Others include Brain abscess, Tremor, Cranial nerve deficits, and seizures are the symptoms of listerial infection in the Central nervous system. 20-50% of the fatality rate of listeriosis has been reported in persons whose immune system is compromised. Neonatal Listeria causes sepsis, pneumonia, meningitis, fever, respiratory distress, jaundice, rash, or lethargy. The symptoms of listeriosis in pregnancy are abortion, septicemia, neonatal death, and meningitis [5].

Patients who take steroids or are suffering from HIV or diabetes are at more risk of infection. Corticosteroids using or Immuno-suppressed pregnant women experience a greater risk of listeriosis as compared with normal pregnant women. Severe maternal illness is caused by an infection in patients with co-morbidities [6].

DIAGNOSIS

Culturing the organism from blood, spinal fluid or amniotic fluid is the way to diagnose infection of Listeria. In diagnosis cultures such as stool and vagina are not useful because some patients do not have the clinical disease and are carriers of the disease [6]. About 1% to 15% population of Listeria has fecal carriage. 33% of cases of Gram stain are helpful because it is intracellular and it resembles diphtheroids, pneumococcal or *Haemophilus* species.

MANAGEMENT

Many antibiotics are active against the organism, ampicillin can be used alone or it can be given in combination with gentamycin. Some patients are given alternative therapies due to allergic reasons or disease state. Secondly, after penicillin, fluoroquinolones, trimethoprim/ sulfamethoxazole, vancomycin, and erythromycin are used. Cephalosporins are not active in the treatment or against Listeria [7]. MIC determination is often used as the basis to predict the efficacy of antibiotics. *Listeria* is *in vitro* susceptible to many antibiotics except the two which are fosfomycin and Cephalosporin. However, a poor clinical outcome is reported. This can occur because the bactericidal mechanisms are refractory for *Listeriae* of many antibiotics, especially ampicillin-amoxicillin. By adding gentamycin a synergism can occur [8]. Some *Listeriae* reside and multiply in the host cells and protected from antibiotics, while some Listeriae penetrates and reaches the cytosol. Most Listeriae remain outside the cell and are easily accessible to the antibiotics which can cross the blood-CSF barrier. In the murine model, Listeria monocytogenes are found in parenchyma cells of liver and spleen and are not easily accessible to many drugs, like gentamycin and penicillin. The effectiveness and therapeutic success of the drugs are dependent upon the models which are being used. Thus, for example, the synergistic effect of gentamycin+ampicillin is found in the model of rabbit meningitis but is not found in the model of the mouse. In the Immuno-compromised host, therapy with antibiotics is not such satisfactory because 30% of deaths are reported with listeriosis [9]. Other alternatives must be used for prevention of the infection and therapy. Defensins are endogenous antibiotics and highly susceptible to *Listeria*. Bacteriocins are bactericidal and are produced by bacterial species, such as enterococci and lactobacilli. However, the use of these alternative measures is not yet feasible. Antibiotics are mainly used in the treatment of Listeriosis which includes: Amoxicillin Penicillin, and Ampicillin [10]. These drugs cannot penetrate intracellularly and they block many PBRs. Under natural conditions, *Listeria* resistance to penicillin is not yet found [10]. For placenta and umbilical cord penetration usually, high doses are used for the surety. In treatment regimens, synergistic effects are found when gentamycin is added and is suggested by *in vitro* studies and animals did not show synergetic effect. Treatment of trimethoprim/sulfamethoxazole (TMP/SMX) is given as alternate to patients who have allergies with using penicillin. Vancomycin is also used for listerial infection. In pregnancy, erythromycin is used to treat listeriosis. Erythromycin rifampin, linezolid, and meropenem are the antibiotics that can also be used in the treatment of listeriosis [10].

REFERENCES

[1] Schlech WF III, Lavigne PM, Bortolussi RA, *et al.* Epidemic listeriosis--evidence for transmission by food. N Engl J Med 1983; 308(4): 203-6.
[http://dx.doi.org/10.1056/NEJM198301273080407] [PMID: 6401354]

[2] Hächler H, Marti G, Giannini P, *et al.* Outbreak of listerosis due to imported cooked ham, Switzerland 2011. Euro Surveill 2013; 18(18): 20469.
[PMID: 23725774]

[3] Cheung VY, Sirkin WL. Listeriosis complicating pregnancy. CMAJ 2009; 181(11): 821-2.
[http://dx.doi.org/10.1503/cmaj.090395] [PMID: 19786466]

[4] Lamont RF, Sobel J, Mazaki-Tovi S, *et al.* Listeriosis in human pregnancy: a systematic review. J Perinat Med 2011; 39(3): 227-36.
[http://dx.doi.org/10.1515/jpm.2011.035] [PMID: 21517700]

[5] Swaminathan B, Gerner-Smidt P. The epidemiology of human listeriosis. Microbes Infect 2007; 9(10): 1236-43.
[http://dx.doi.org/10.1016/j.micinf.2007.05.011] [PMID: 17720602]

[6] Janakiraman V. Listeriosis in pregnancy: diagnosis, treatment, and prevention. Rev Obstet Gynecol 2008; 1(4): 179-85.
[PMID: 19173022]

[7] Hof H, Nichterlein T, Kretschmar M. Management of listeriosis. Clin Microbiol Rev 1997; 10(2): 345-57.
[http://dx.doi.org/10.1128/CMR.10.2.345] [PMID: 9105758]

[8] Charpentier E, Gerbaud G, Jacquet C, Rocourt J, Courvalin P. Incidence of antibiotic resistance in Listeria species. J Infect Dis 1995; 172(1): 277-81.
[http://dx.doi.org/10.1093/infdis/172.1.277] [PMID: 7797931]

[9] Slifman NR, Gershon SK, Lee JH, Edwards ET, Braun MM. Listeria monocytogenes infection as a complication of treatment with tumor necrosis factor α-neutralizing agents. Arthritis Rheum 2003; 48(2): 319-24.
[http://dx.doi.org/10.1002/art.10758] [PMID: 12571839]

[10] Temple ME, Nahata MC. Treatment of listeriosis. Ann Pharmacother 2000; 34(5): 656-61.
[http://dx.doi.org/10.1345/aph.19315] [PMID: 10852095]

CHAPTER 35

Bacterial Meningitis: An Inflammation of Meninges by Bacteria

Muhammad Imran Qadir[*] and **Irtiqa Masood**

Institute of Molecular Biology & Biotechnology, Bahauddin Zakariya University, Multan, Pakistan

Abstract: Meningitis is the inflammation of the membrane of meninges that is caused by a different microorganism. Bacterial meningitis is a lethal disease with the mortality rate in older adults is <20%. The bacteria start to replicate in the cerebrospinal fluid CSF and meninges and then infection takes place. It causes fever, headache, nausea, photophobia, vomiting, nuchal rigidity with complications of arthritis and hydrocephalus. *Streptococcus pneumoniae* is the main cause of bacterial meningitis in older children. Different laboratory diagnosis like antigen screening, gram staining is used to test bacterial meningitis and antibiotics like chloramphenicol, gentamicin, tobramycin, second and third-generation cephalosporin, metronidazole, and rifampin are used against different bacterial microorganisms. Vaccines are available for 23 serotypes of *Streptococcus pneumoniae*.

Keywords: Antibiotics, Bacterial meningitis, Inflammation of CSF, *Streptococcus pneumoniae*.

INTRODUCTION

Meningitis is a disease that causes infection in the cerebrospinal fluid (CSF) in which the membrane surrounding the brain and spinal cord get inflamed. It is mainly caused by several bacteria, fungi, and viruses. In neonates, the fatality rate is high as compared to infants [1]. Bacteria from *group B streptococci* cause meningitis in premature babies and this disease starts to appear in the second week of life. Gram-negative bacteria including *E. coli* are also responsible for bacterial meningitis in newborn babies in developing countries [2]. In older children, meningitis is caused by the *Streptococcus pneumoniae* and *Neisseria meningitides*. *Streptococcus pneumoniae* contains 84 serotypes of which 1, 3, 4, 7-11 serotypes are responsible for most of the diseases. Tuberculosis meningitis is more prevalent in people with a high risk of tuberculosis [3, 4]. Other causes of

[*] **Corresponding author Muhammad Imran Qadir:** Institute of Molecular Biology and Biotechnology, Bahauddin Zakariya University, Multan, Pakistan; Tel: +92-61-9210071; Ext. 1920; Fax: +92-61-9210068; E-mail: mrimranqadir@hotmail.com

Muhammad Imran Qadir (Ed.)
All rights reserved-© 2020 Bentham Science Publishers

viral meningitis include mumps virus, the varicella-zoster virus, enterovirus, and HIV. The Herpes simplex virus is responsible to cause Mollaret's meningitis [5]. Meningitis caused by fungi contains *Candida* species, *Coccidioides immitis* [6]. According to the Centre for Disease Control and Prevention (CDC) study bacterial meningitis is increased by *Listeria monocytogenes*, gram-negative bacilli, *Streptococcus pneumoniae*, and *Streptococcus agalactiae.*

Bacterial pathogens enter into the CSF and meninges *via* local invasion and hematogenous spread. Bacterial starts to replicate rapidly once it gains entry to the CSF or meninges and it activates the inflammatory response that leads to neuronal apoptosis, vasogenic edema, and high intracranial pressure that results in cerebral infarction, cortical vein thrombosis, and empyema leading to stroke syndromes, coma, and death [7].

SYMPTOMS

The symptoms of the bacterial meningitis are fever and chills, confusion, photophobia, nuchal rigidity (stiffness of the neck), headache, consciousness level changes, swelling of the eyes (papilledema), petechial rashes on the skin, nausea, and vomiting leading to complication like central nervous system CNS with the increased WBC count, arthritis and hydrocephalus [8 - 11].

LABORATORY DIAGNOSIS

For the diagnosis of bacterial meningitis, CSF must be examined thoroughly. Cultures of the CFS are used. Lumbar puncture (LP) is used for the diagnosis of bacterial meningitis. LP assesses red blood cell, white blood cell WBC count, glucose, opening pressure, and proteins. But with herniation LP is not suitable to use. Computerized tomography CT scan is used before LP. Abnormal CT scan shows abnormal visual fields, aphasia, abnormal consciousness level, leg and arm drift, confusion in giving answers. As well as Gram staining is also used. In the untreated bacterial meningitis, the gram stain result is positive. Bacterial meningitis causes increased WBC count, hypoglycorrhachia, neutrophilic predominance. Bacterial antigen testing is also available for *E. coli*, *S. pneumoniae, H. influenza*. Polymerase chain reaction PCR involves bacterial primers that are highly conserved and is under investigation [3, 12].

MANAGEMENT

Bactericidal antibiotics are used to prevent bacterial replication in CSF and meninges. Penicillin G with a dose of 20-24 million units is used for *S. pneumoniae*. Ampicillin 12g with gentamicin, tobramycin 5mg/kg is used against *Listeria monocytogenes*. Cefotaxime 8-12g or ceftriaxone 4-6g is used for

Haemophilus influenza, Enterobacteriaceae, and *Streptococcus pneumoniae*. For *Staphylococcus aureus* that is methicillin-sensitive nafcillin 8-12g is used and for methicillin-resistant vancomycin 2g is used [12]. Some antibiotics have excellent penetration into CSF, some have bad penetration according to [12, 13] as described in Table **3**.

Table 3. Penetration of antibiotics in CSF.

Excellent penetration	Good penetration	Negligible penetration
Metronidazole	Penicillin	Tobramycin
Chloramphenicol	Third-generation cephalosporin	Gentamicin
Trimethoprim-sulphamethoxazole	Vancomycin	A most first and second-generation cephalosporin
Rifampin	Cefuroxime	Aminoglycosides

Several bacterial meningitis diseases are caused by *Streptococcus pneumonia* [13]. One-third of the people have received the pneumococcal vaccine and the rate is higher in older adults. There is a reduction seen in the pneumococcal disease when conjugated *Streptococcus pneumoniae* vaccine is given to the recipients. Vaccines are currently available for 23 serotypes of *Streptococcus pneumonia*. An improved pneumococcal vaccine is a major goal. The individuals that have had serious infections with *Neisseria meningitidis*, for those vaccines are recommended [13].

CONSENT FOR PUBLICATION

Not applicable.

CONFLICT OF INTEREST

The authors declare no conflict of interest, financial or otherwise.

ACKNOWLEDGEMENTS

Declared none.

REFERENCES

[1]   Sáez-Llorens X, McCracken GH Jr. Bacterial meningitis in children. Lancet 2003; 361(9375): 2139-48.
        [http://dx.doi.org/10.1016/S0140-6736(03)13693-8] [PMID: 12826449]

[2]   Moreno MT, Vargas S, Poveda R, Sáez-Llorens X. Neonatal sepsis and meningitis in a developing Latin American country. Pediatr Infect Dis J 1994; 13(6): 516-20.
        [PMID: 8078740]

[3]   Tunkel AR, Hartman BJ, Kaplan SL, *et al.* Practice guidelines for the management of bacterial meningitis. Clin Infect Dis 2004; 39(9): 1267-84.
[http://dx.doi.org/10.1086/425368] [PMID: 15494903]

[4]   Thwaites G, Chau TT, Mai NT, Drobniewski F, McAdam K, Farrar J. Tuberculous meningitis. J Neurol Neurosurg Psychiatry 2000; 68(3): 289-99.
[http://dx.doi.org/10.1136/jnnp.68.3.289] [PMID: 10675209]

[5]   Logan SA, MacMahon E. Viral meningitis. BMJ 2008; 336(7634): 36-40.
[http://dx.doi.org/10.1136/bmj.39409.673657.AE] [PMID: 18174598]

[6]   Boehm S. Clinical neurology of the older adult. Clinical Neurology 2016; 1

[7]   Ellerin TB, Tunkel AR. Acute bacterial meningitis. 2004.

[8]   van de Beek D, de Gans J, Spanjaard L, Weisfelt M, Reitsma JB, Vermeulen M. Clinical features and prognostic factors in adults with bacterial meningitis. N Engl J Med 2004; 351(18): 1849-59.
[http://dx.doi.org/10.1056/NEJMoa040845] [PMID: 15509818]

[9]   Gorse GJ, Thrupp LD, Nudleman KL, Wyle FA, Hawkins B, Cesario TC. Bacterial meningitis in the elderly. Arch Intern Med 1984; 144(8): 1603-7.
[http://dx.doi.org/10.1001/archinte.1984.00350200107016] [PMID: 6466018]

[10]   Behrman RE, Meyers BR, Mendelson MH, Sacks HS, Hirschman SZ. Central nervous system infections in the elderly. Arch Intern Med 1989; 149(7): 1596-9.
[http://dx.doi.org/10.1001/archinte.1989.00390070112017] [PMID: 2568111]

[11]   *E. coli.* Bacterial meningitis 1992.

[12]   Choi C. Bacterial Meningitis and Brain Abscess Infectious Disease in the Aging. Springer 2009; pp. 181-99.

[13]   Choi C. Bacterial meningitis Infectious Disease in the Aging. Springer 2001; pp. 113-24.
[http://dx.doi.org/10.1007/978-1-59259-026-1_11]

CHAPTER 36

Nosocomial Infections: Hospital Acquired Infections

Muhammad Imran Qadir[*] and **Mahreen Fatima**

Institute of Molecular Biology & Biotechnology, Bahauddin Zakariya University, Multan, Pakistan

Abstract: The term nosocomial can apply to that type of a disease that is acquired by a patient when he is under medical care. These types of infections are also known as HAI grow into patients when he stays at the hospital and taken supplementary types of medical facilities. It can be appeared in both cases either during hospitalization or after the time of discharge. Pathogens which are a major basis of such infections are called nosocomial pathogens. Worldwide, in healthcare systems, urinary tract infections are the most common complications. According to recent data, 30% of Nosocomial infections related to UT are caused by gram-negative bacteria.

KeyWords: Hospital-Acquired Infections, UTIs.

INTRODUCTION

"Nosocomial" and "hospital-acquired" are synonymous with each other and this type of infection has been caught in a hospital and most organisms that show resistance to antibiotics are responsible for it and acquired in any healthcare centre when patient management is related to it [1]. In two-third, the cases the origin of Nosocomial infection is acquired by the patients in any healthcare institution which are not present in patients being admitted hospital. After review of literature completed by using the Medical Literature Analysis and PubMed, we can define the nosocomial urinary tract infections as, "An infection in any part of our urinary system *i.e.* kidneys, urethra, bladders, and ureters". The urethra and bladder are a big source of lower urinary tract Nosocomial infection and greater risk of disease in women than men [2].

The second most common UTI is caused by gram-negative bacilli which affect humans throughout their lifetime. Gram-negative bacteria are a major cause of

[*] **Corresponding author Muhammad Imran Qadir:** Institute of Molecular Biology and Biotechnology, Bahauddin Zakariya University, Multan, Pakistan; Tel: +92-61-9210071; Ext. 1920; Fax: +92-61-9210068; E-mail: mrimranqadir@hotmail.com

Muhammad Imran Qadir (Ed.)
All rights reserved-© 2020 Bentham Science Publishers

wound or surgical sight infection because these bacteria are resistant multi drugs and antibiotics [3]. These bacteria are responsible for nosocomial infections with increasing frequency. The major causes of uti occur when gram-negative bacilli enter the urinary tract urethra and later start to multiply in the bladder.

Currently available antibiotics for increasing pathogenicity of bacterial infections are limited in numbers. This issue is especially for gram-negative nosocomial UTIs "centers for disease control and prevention (CDC)" reveal threats about gram-negative bacilli to develop drug-resistant and scarceness of coming treatments to fight organisms. Most types of nosocomial uti infections gram-negative bacilli may have the capacity to cause infection and a very large number of bacteria responsible for uti. In this way, rehabilitation investigation for the nosocomial infection that is measurable control of Proteus rettgeri, serratia marcescens, and Klebsiella pneumoniae. These three organisms are responsible for seven outbreaks.

Pseudomonas that mostly causes nosocomial multidrug-resistant infection but here is not investigating any outbreaks. A general acceptance of confrontation to antibiotics is a characteristic of such pathogen that may reflect the capacity of pseudomonas to cause epidemic infrequently although slide variation on a single pattern of antimicrobial sensitivity outbreak. The variation in drug sensitivity serotype and biochemical markers of stains chemicals. For these multi-resistant pathogens hospitalize patients were the primary reservoir. Uti went unrecognized in all of these outbreaks contributed to the reservoir. For these pathogens, not other environmental reservoir thought to be an important source and in any of outbreaks no common source identified was found but medical equipment may culture-positive such as cart tops, sink drains, and bed railings. It is suggested by an epidemiologic investigation that in all seven outbreaks organisms were transmitted from one patient to another patient on the hand of a person. Urinary catheterization and exposure to broad-spectrum antimicrobial therapy multidrug-resistant strain are more common factors that exposed hospitalized patients to urinary infection.

Nosocomial infections are increasing day by day with advancement in antimicrobial agents and life-saving methodologies which expose a patient to the disease. Despite using control health care measurements, nosocomial infections are associated with mortality and morbidity. Several hospital-acquired infections are increase which may respond in adding extra health care expenses and cause an economic crisis. In the hospital environment, this problem becomes more complicated when treating multidrug-resistant (MDR) microorganisms. Mostly in the hospitalized patient, infection is caused by different pathogens.

In most nosocomial infections gram-negative bacteria are responsible *i.e.* gram-negative bacilli. Some extrinsic and intrinsic factors are more common to affect hospitalized patients by these pathogens. Although nosocomial infections uti by gram-negative bacilli are not avoidable the use of hygienic hospital methodology and standard practices may reduce such nosocomial infection at a significant level.

TYPES OF NOSOCOMIAL INFECTION

There are 50 potentially specific infection sites for surveillance out of 13 major types of healthcare-associated infection sites according to clinical and biological criteria. Surgical wounds and other soft tissue infections, urinary tract infection, respiratory infection, gastroenteritis, and meningitis are the most common types of nosocomial infections caused by gram-negative bacteria [4]. Types of nosocomial urinary infections have been changed due to an increased number of invasive procedures for therapeutic and diagnostic purposes [5].

The Anticipation of Gram-Negative Nosocomial Urinary Tract Infection

In health care, everyone including staff and individuals is equally responsible for the prevention of anticipation of gram-negative nosocomial urinary tract infection. For patients and organizations to reduce the risk of infection everyone must work cooperatively. However, all hospital infections are not curable but with the struggle, many uti nosocomial infections can be prevented.

The most common anticipation toward infection is frequent hand washing and to wear gloves, masks, and gown but the cost will be unnecessarily increased due to inappropriate use of these. Although poor hygiene practices are done by the staff in the area of the hospital may be responsible factors for vectors of disease and virulent gram-negative bacilli are spread in their patients and exposed difficulties to control uti infections.

Agents of Nosocomial Urinary Tract Infection

Any microbe could have the capability to cause infection but the specific organism is responsible for a large number of hospital infection in hospitalized patients almost 90 percent nosocomial urinary tract infection are caused by bacteria, some are mycobacterial, fungal or viral but some agents are less commonly involved like protozoal [1]. The most common type of gram-negative bacilli is Pseudomonas (P.) aeruginosa, Legionella, and some other members of the Enterobacteriaceae family *i.e.Escherichia* (*E.coli*), Proteus mirabilis, *Salmonella* spp., Serratia marcescens and Klebsiella pneumonia [6]. *Escherichia* (*E.coli*), S. aureus, and *P. aeruginosa* are the most frequently reported nosocomial pathogens.

BACTERIOLOGY OF COMMONLY ISOLATED NOSOCOMIAL UTI PATHOGENS

1. *Pseudomonas Aeruginosa*

P. aeruginosa is mucoid gram-negative which is arranged in pairs of polysaccharide capsule. *P. aeruginosa* is a major cause of urinary tract infections. Their identification is done by their colonial characteristic and biochemical tests. In respiratory and gastrointestinal tracts of hospitalized patients they may be transiently colonized, especially when the patient is treated by broad-spectrum drugs, hospitalized periods, and exposed to therapy equipment .when the normal defense mechanism is impaired, the pathogenesis due to these organisms is started. For example, direct tissue damage occurs when body barriers are disrupted as in urinary catheter. In this way, bacteria invade locally by making colonies in the membrane and responsible for systematic urinary tract diseases. Different virulent factors and toxins are involved to mediate the processes *i.e.* enzymes, pili [7].

2. *Escherichia Coli*

E.coli is an oxidase negative, anaerobic and gram-negative bacteria. It involves endotoxin-induced shock and belongs to gram-negative species. By this organism, different types of diseases occur in immune-compromised nosocomial patients *i.e.* pneumonia, meningitis, diarrheal disease, and wound infections. Urinary tract infections are one of the major diseases which is caused by these organisms in hospitalized patients. Enterobacteriaceae family related to *E. coli* possesses very wide ranges of virulence factors (antimicrobial-resistant, endotoxin, capsule, antigenic phase variation). For UTIs disease, some *E.coli* strains are responsible for specialized virulence factors. *E.coli* cause more uti infections as compared to other organisms as shown in

SOURCES AND TERMINATION OF INFECTIONS

Usually directed or from time to time circuitously by way of secretion from the body, contact is a very much important pathway by which nosocomial urinary tract infections are transmitted. For Food born and water-borne infections, the faeco-oral route is the verge of entry. Oropharynx, the gastrointestinal tract, and the urinary tract are the most frequent reservoirs used for nosocomial colonies.

RISK FACTORS FOR NOSOCOMIAL URINARY TRACT INFECTIONS

There are two categories of factors that cause infections. One is an intrinsic factor and the other is extrinsic. Hospitalized patients are exposed to infections because of different risk factors and these factors cause various reasons for infections [8]. When patient acquired infections due to underlying disease conditions are called intrinsic risk factors and when patient care staff or institute is responsible for disease in patients is called extrinsic risk factors. Nosocomial urinary tract infections are extrinsic and these factors occur frequently in medical centers during the use of invasive devices and surgical operations, immunosuppressive agents, use of broad-spectrum antibiotics, and also by gram-negative bacteria. Some other important factors that are responsible for nosocomial infections are patient's age, old diseases like diabetes, and tumors [9].

MODIFICATION OF RISK FACTOR AND SURVEILLANCE

The care of indwelling urinary catheters should be reviewed with all personnel which is the criteria of catheterization. Patients who need catheter drainage, the significance of maintaining a blocked drainage system should be emphasized [10]. The anti-microbial agent ought to be appropriately stressed out while using broad-spectrum antibiotics. However, a narrow spectrum should be used as an alternative drug where it is possible. For the amendment of prescribing practices, the restriction of antibiotic uses should be taken as consideration.

In surveillance, early achievement is to recognize risk factors and allow them to measures the cause of infection [11]. A degree of compliance with suggested control measures and to assess the effectiveness to detect the new infection a new means for inspection should be established. In an epidemic situation which consign patients at soaring threat of infection, should monitor specific patient-care procedure by a surveillance officer [6].

CONCLUSION

In short, urinary tract infections epidemics with multidrug-resistant pathogens (gram-negative bacilli) are responsible for factors that cause overall nosocomial infections. There are many difficulties to control them. But here is a hope that guidelines by this review will be provided successful approaches to control the problem.

CONSENT FOR PUBLICATION

Not applicable.

CONFLICT OF INTEREST

The authors declare no conflict of interest, financial or otherwise.

ACKNOWLEDGEMENTS

Declared none.

REFERENCES

[1]　Bereket W, Hemalatha K, Getenet B, *et al.* Update on bacterial nosocomial infections. Eur Rev Med Pharmacol Sci 2012; 16(8): 1039-44.
[PMID: 22913154]

[2]　Chikere C, Omoni V, Chikere B. Distribution of potential nosocomial pathogens in a hospital environment. Afr J Biotechnol 2008; 7(20)

[3]　Emori TG, Gaynes RP. An overview of nosocomial infections, including the role of the microbiology laboratory. Clin Microbiol Rev 1993; 6(4): 428-42.
[http://dx.doi.org/10.1128/CMR.6.4.428] [PMID: 8269394]

[4]　Raka L, Zoutman D, Mulliqi G, *et al.* Prevalence of nosocomial infections in high-risk units in the university clinical center of Kosova. Infect Control Hosp Epidemiol 2006; 27(4): 421-3.
[http://dx.doi.org/10.1086/503387] [PMID: 16622824]

[5]　Duque ÂS, Ferreira AF, Cezário RC, Gontijo Filho PP. Nosocomial infections in two hospitals in Uberlandia, Brazil Rev panam infectol 2007; 9(4): 8-14.

[6]　McGowan JE Jr, Finland M. Usage of antibiotics in a general hospital: effect of requiring justification. J Infect Dis 1974; 130(2): 165-8.
[http://dx.doi.org/10.1093/infdis/130.2.165] [PMID: 4842338]

[7]　Contreras GA, DiazGranados CA, Cortes L, *et al.* Nosocomial outbreak of *Enteroccocus gallinarum*: untaming of rare species of enterococci. J Hosp Infect 2008; 70(4): 346-52.
[http://dx.doi.org/10.1016/j.jhin.2008.07.012] [PMID: 18799242]

[8]　Murray PR, Rosenthal KS, Pfaller MA. Medical microbiology 2015.

[9]　Lahsaeizadeh S, Jafari H, Askarian M. Healthcare-associated infection in Shiraz, Iran 2004-2005. J Hosp Infect 2008; 69(3): 283-7.
[http://dx.doi.org/10.1016/j.jhin.2008.05.006] [PMID: 18550217]

[10]　Schaberg DR, Weinstein RA, Stamm WE. Epidemics of nosocomial urinary tract infection caused by multiply resistant gram-negative bacilli: epidemiology and control. J Infect Dis 1976; 133(3): 363-6.
[http://dx.doi.org/10.1093/infdis/133.3.363] [PMID: 768384]

[11]　Kunin CM, Tupasi T, Craig WA. Use of antibiotics. A brief exposition of the problem and some tentative solutions. Ann Intern Med 1973; 79(4): 555-60.
[http://dx.doi.org/10.7326/0003-4819-79-4-555] [PMID: 4795880]

CHAPTER 37

*Campylobacter*iosis: A Food Borne Illness Caused by *Campylobacter*

Muhammad Imran Qadir[*] and **Zunaira Akhtar**

Institute of Molecular Biology & Biotechnology, Bahauddin Zakariya University, Multan, Pakistan

Abstract: *Campylobacter*iosis is a foodborne illness caused by *Campylobacter* (*C. jejuni*), gram-negative bacteria, which cause diarrhea and other symptoms like fever pain and cramps. It transmits from food spoilage, untreated water, raw milk containing the bacteria, contact with pets, and farm animals having diarrhea. Person to person transmission is uncommon. It can be diagnosed by different techniques like the culture of bacteria taken from the bloody stool is the way for culture, molecular methods like a polymerase chain reaction, antigen testing, and DNA microarray. It can be managed by taking different precautionary measures, considering various hygienic rules, and through proper medication like antibiotics. But antibiotics are not preferred to those patients having a weak immune system and AIDS.

Keywords: Antibiotics, *Campylobacter*iosis, Culturing, Diarrhea, Molecular Technique.

INTRODUCTION

*Campylobacter*iosis is caused by *Campylobacter* bacterium (*C. jejuni*). It's a foodborne illness. It is the most common bacterial infection in humans. It causes diarrhea and other serious complications like dysentery syndrome, fever, cramp, pain, and sometimes bloody [1]. *Campylobacter* is a gram-negative, non-spore forming bacteria. It is a comma or spiral shape found in swine, cattle, and birds. It mostly causes diarrhea and other complications if left untreated like tissue damage in the gut. It causes cholera and latent autoimmune effects. The infection clears up in 2-8 days. Every year about 1 million people are infected in the United States. Infants and children have more chance of *Campylobacter*iosis infection than adults. But it can infect at any age and its infection is more severe in summer than in winter.

[*] **Corresponding author Muhammad Imran Qadir:** Institute of Molecular Biology and Biotechnology, Bahauddin Zakariya University, Multan, Pakistan; Tel: +92-61-9210071; Ext. 1920; Fax: +92-61-9210068; E-mail: mrimranqadir@hotmail.com

Muhammad Imran Qadir (Ed.)
All rights reserved-© 2020 Bentham Science Publishers

There are many reasons for the prevalence of this disease. It is caused by eating uncooked food especially uncooked poultry [2]. *Campylobacter* bacteria live in the digestive tract of animals including cattle and poultry, raw milk may have *Campylobacter* bacteria. That bacteria may present in the sewage system and water in developing countries [3], drinking untreated water is the major factor. It can transmit through contact with cats, dogs, and pets with diarrhea. Food from animal origin plays an important role in transmitting *Campylobacter* bacteria to humans. Person to person transmission is not reported. Environmental factors and the wild animal accounts only 3% for this infection and remaining are considered due to chicken and farm animals for meat.

SYMPTOMS

Symptoms include diarrhea, blood in the stool, abdominal pain, cramps, fever, headache, vomit, and malaise. HIV patients are more likely to have severe symptoms like prolonged diarrhea. people may develop Guillain- Barre syndrome in which nerves present between the brain and spinal cord may damage. It only occurs with *C. upsaliensis* and *C. jejuni.*

Some people may not have any symptoms due to the weakened immune system.

DIAGNOSIS

There are various techniques used for the diagnosis of *Campylobacter*iosis.

Culturing Techniques

Obtaining cultures of organisms from a stool sample are always the best way to diagnose this infection. If laboratory facilities are not available then fecal smears dark- field microscopy and gram stain provide the best presumptive diagnosis [4]. The basis of diagnosis is to isolate the bacteria from faeces and basal media are used which include:

- Butzler's media.
- Preston media [5].

The culturing process is carried out at $42\,^\circ$C.

It can also be diagnosed *via* antigen testing EIA and PCR.

PCR Based Assay

Biochemical tests and bacteriological analysis such as culture media and isolation are mostly used for the analysis of different samples but they are time consuming and laborious as well.

PCR is now extensively used as a molecular method for the detection of *Campylobacter*. The widely used PCR are:

- Multiplex PCR [6].
- Real-time PCR [7].

PCR gives more reliable results within no time and gel electrophoresis is used to isolate and DNA sequencing techniques are now used as a molecular basis. New markers may be suggested, but not extensively in use nowadays.

DNA Microarray

This technique is now using as a diagnostic tool.

MANAGEMENT

*Campylobacter*iosis can be managed by taking certain preventive measures, treatments, and other alternatives.

Prevention

World health organization (WHO) recommends the following.

- Food must be hot and properly cooked when served.
- By using boiled water, it can be controlled.
- After contact with pets and farm animals, the hand should be wash properly and frequently [8].
- Pasteurized milk should be used rather than raw milk.
- Fruits and vegetables should be washed before eating.
- Hygienic rules should be followed during food handling food preservation, professionally and at home.
- Contact with farm animals and pets should be avoided.
- Proper tests and treatments must be taken.
- Broiler chicken should be avoided [9].

TREATMENTS

Treatments include the electrolytes and the replacement of fluids. Lots of fluid should be drunk as in case of diarrhea. In the case of dehydration, intravenous fluid and oral fluid are usually prescribed.

Antibiotics

Antibiotics are given when symptoms are severe [10]. Commonly used antibiotic are:

- Ciprofloxin.
- Levofloxacin.
- Azithromycin.
- Erythromycin is frequently used because of its low resistance.

Alternatives

Tetracycline and anti-diarrheal drugs can be used as alternatives.

CONSENT FOR PUBLICATION

Not applicable.

CONFLICT OF INTEREST

The authors declare no conflict of interest, financial or otherwise.

ACKNOWLEDGEMENTS

Declared none.

REFERENCES

[1]   Coker AO, Isokpehi RD, Thomas BN, Amisu KO, Obi CL. Human *Campylobacter*iosis in developing countries. Emerg Infect Dis 2002; 8(3): 237-44.
        [http://dx.doi.org/10.3201/eid0803.010233] [PMID: 11927019]

[2]   Wingstrand A, Neimann J, Engberg J, *et al.* Fresh chicken as main risk factor for *Campylobacter*iosis, Denmark. Emerg Infect Dis 2006; 12(2): 280-5.
        [http://dx.doi.org/10.3201/eid1202.050936] [PMID: 16494755]

[3]   Wilson DJ, Gabriel E, Leatherbarrow AJ, *et al.* Tracing the source of *Campylobacter*iosis. PLoS Genet 2008; 4(9)e1000203
        [http://dx.doi.org/10.1371/journal.pgen.1000203] [PMID: 18818764]

[4]   Arnold ME, Jones EM, Lawes JR, *et al.* Bayesian analysis of culture and PCR methods for detection of *Campylobacter* spp. in broiler caecal samples. Epidemiol Infect 2015; 143(2): 298-307.
        [http://dx.doi.org/10.1017/S0950268814000454] [PMID: 24650797]

[5]   Keramas G, Bang DD, Lund M, *et al.* Use of culture, PCR analysis, and DNA microarrays for detection of *Campylobacter* jejuni and *Campylobacter* coli from chicken feces. J Clin Microbiol 2004; 42(9): 3985-91.
[http://dx.doi.org/10.1128/JCM.42.9.3985-3991.2004] [PMID: 15364980]

[6]   Khan IUH, Cloutier M, Libby M, Lapen DR, Wilkes G, Topp E. Enhanced Single-tube Multiplex PCR Assay for Detection and Identification of Six Arcobacter Species. J Appl Microbiol 2017; 123(6): 1522-32.
[http://dx.doi.org/10.1111/jam.13597] [PMID: 28960631]

[7]   de Boer P, Rahaoui H, Leer RJ, Montijn RC, van der Vossen JM. Real-time PCR detection of *Campylobacter spp.*: A comparison to classic culturing and enrichment. Food Microbiol 2015; 51: 96-100.
[http://dx.doi.org/10.1016/j.fm.2015.05.006] [PMID: 26187833]

[8]   Wagenaar JA, Newell DG, Kalupahana RS, Mughini-Gras L. Campylobacter: animal reservoirs, human infections, and options for control Zoonoses-infections affecting humans and animals. Springer 2015; pp. 159-77.
[http://dx.doi.org/10.1007/978-94-017-9457-2_6]

[9]   Umaraw P, Prajapati A, Verma AK, Pathak V, Singh VP. Control of *Campylobacter* in poultry industry from farm to poultry processing unit: A review. Crit Rev Food Sci Nutr 2017; 57(4): 659-65.
[http://dx.doi.org/10.1080/10408398.2014.935847] [PMID: 25898290]

[10]   Hussein K, Raz-Pasteur A, Shachor-Meyouhas Y, *et al. Campylobacter bacteraemia*: 16 years of experience in a single centre. Infect Dis (Lond) 2016; 48(11-12): 796-9.
[http://dx.doi.org/10.1080/23744235.2016.1195916] [PMID: 27320494]

CHAPTER 38

Brucellosis: Undulant Fever, Malta Fever, Gibraltar Fever or Bang's Disease

Muhammad Imran Qadir[*] and **Afia Javaid**

Institute of Molecular Biology & Biotechnology, Bahauddin Zakariya University, Multan, Pakistan

Abstract: Brucellosis is an infectious disease caused by the species of bacteria *Brucella*. Animals are the primary host for bacteria; they are transferred from animals to humans (secondary host) by eating undercooked meat and unpasteurized dairy products. The symptom for brucellosis varies from mild like simple flu, fever, headache to acute like tissue and dysfunction of organs. Due to its complicated symptoms, the diagnosis of brucellosis is difficult but blood and bone marrow samples are still used for its diagnosis. Different techniques like culturing, molecular methods, and serological tests are used for its diagnosis. Antibiotics are used to prevent relapses and to minimize their symptoms. Antibiotics alone or the combination of two are used for the treatment of brucellosis. Other precautionary measures like safety and hygienic conditions should be considered to prevent disease.

Keywords: Antibiotics, Brucella, Culturing & Molecular Techniques, Polymorphonuclear Cells, Lymph Nodes.

INTRODUCTION

Brucellosis is an infectious disease also known as undulant fever, Malta fever, Gibraltar fever, and Bang's disease. It is caused by bacteria brucella which is aerobic, rod-shaped (coccobacillus) gram-negative, non-motile, and non-spore forming bacteria [1]. Brucellosis spread from animals to humans by direct fluid contacts like blood or tissue fluid, eating uncooked meat, unpasteurized milk, and dairy products like cheese [2]. Different types of stains infect different types of animals like cattle is infected by Brucella abortus, sheep and goats infected by *Brucella melitensis*, pigs, sheep, dogs, wood desert rats are infected by Brucella suis, *Brucella ovis*, *Brucella canis*, and *Brucella neotomae* respectively [3]. Brucella infects almost all domestic animals excluding cats which are resistant to

[*] **Corresponding author Muhammad Imran Qadir:** Institute of Molecular Biology and Biotechnology, Bahauddin Zakariya University, Multan, Pakistan; Tel: +92-61-9210071; Ext. 1920; Fax: +92-61-9210068; E-mail: mrimranqadir@hotmail.com

Muhammad Imran Qadir (Ed.)
All rights reserved-© 2020 Bentham Science Publishers

bacteria brucella. The disease is very old from a Roman era, it is detected in carbonized cheese [4]. The prevalence of brucellosis in Colombia is between 2.4 to 5%, in Tanzania 3.5% and in northern Tanzania 8% [5]. The cases of the prevalence of brucellosis in Asia, Africa, Latin America, and the middle east are 10 per 100 000 population and 100 per 100 000 cases are seen in Saudi Arabia, Jordan, Iraq, middle east, and the Mediterranean rim. The prevalence of brucellosis also depends on factors like the trade of animals, husbandry practices, and preparation of food. Brucella is taken by macrophages and polymorphonuclear cells within which bacteria replicate and survive then they move to blood circulation and lymph nodes and settled into various organs and tissues. According to the world health organization (WHO), a half million people each year in 100 countries were infected by brucellosis. Humans are the secondary and indirect host for this disease, but the primary hosts are domestic animals. Besides a zoonotic problem, it is also bioterrorism of category B.

SYMPTOMS

Its symptoms vary from mild to acute.

- Recurrent fever
- Fatigue
- Headache
- Myalgia
- Weightloss
- Arthralgia
- Anorexia
- Pain in muscles, joints
- Night sweats [2].

Other Complications

In some cases, brucellosis also affects organ systems like:

- Hematological system (causing anemia, leucopenia, and thrombocytopenia)
- Neurological system (causing
- meningitis, neuritis and encephalitis)
- A Genitourinary system (causing orchitis and epididymitis)
- A Pulmonary system (causing bronchitis, empyema and pneumonitis)

Death is very rare in case of brucellosis, only 2% of cases of death are reported in acute conditions [6].

DIAGNOSIS

Human brucellosis, clinical features overlap with many other infectious and noninfectious diseases, therefore its diagnosis is problematic. However, blood samples, bone marrow samples and other body fluids are used for the diagnosis of brucellosis. A Blood test for antibodies detection against *brucella* bacteria is also used. Different techniques are used to test these samples which are molecular-based methods, serological tests and culturing [7].

Molecular Based Methods

- PCR based assays.
- Standard PCR.
- Real-time PCR.
- Nested and semi-nested PCR.
- A Multiple locus VNTR analysis.
- Loop-mediated isothermal amplification assay.

Culturing Techniques

- Conventional culture technique.
- Semi-automated blood culture technique.
- Lysis centrifugation blood culture technique.

Serological Test

- Serum agglutination test.
- Rose Bengal test.
- Lateral flow assay.
- Enzyme-linked immunosorbent assay (ELISA).
- An Immunocapture agglutination test.
- Coombs antiglobulin agglutination test [8].
- Complement fixation test.

TREATMENT

Different types of antibiotics are used for the treatment of brucelloses like rifampicin, chloramphenicol, tetracycline, streptomycin, trimethoprim-sulfamethoxazole, quinolones, doxycycline and gentamicin. They may be used separately or a combination of two may also be used. For patients with acute brucellosis combination of doxycycline along with rifampicin or tetracycline is used [9]. Another method used for the treatment of brucellosis is the addition of hydroxychloroquine with doxycycline and streptomycin this method is very effective because it reduces the relapses of disease and helps improving its clinical symptoms [10]. It may take a few weeks to several months to recover from the disease and it depends on the type of bacteria and the severity of diseases. No vaccine is available for brucellosis.

PREVENTION

Prevention from brucellosis is possible by taking the following measures:

- By not eating the undercooked meat.
- By not using the unpasteurized dairy products like milk, cheese, *etc*
- Persons like butchers, slaughterhouse workers, veterinarians who deal with animals must wear gloves and aprons so that they may not get infected by direct contact (broken or damaged skin).
- People who work with animal tissues and fluids like laboratory workers must use protective clothing, masks and they should work under BSL3.
- Contact with pets should be avoided.
- In case of skin injuries contact with animals should be avoided as bacteria may transmit from animal to human.

CONSENT FOR PUBLICATION

Not applicable.

CONFLICT OF INTEREST

The authors declare no conflict of interest, financial or otherwise.

ACKNOWLEDGEMENTS

Declared none.

REFERENCES

[1]   Russell-Lodrigue KE, Killeen SZ, Ficht TA, Roy CJ. Mucosal bacterial dissemination in a rhesus macaque model of experimental brucellosis. J Med Primatol 2018; 47(1): 75-7.
[http://dx.doi.org/10.1111/jmp.12282] [PMID: 28573738]

[2]   Cossaboom CM, Kharod GA, Salzer JS, *et al.* Notes from the Field: Brucella abortus Vaccine Strain RB51 Infection and Exposures Associated with Raw Milk Consumption - Wise County, Texas, 2017. MMWR Morb Mortal Wkly Rep 2018; 67(9): 286.
[http://dx.doi.org/10.15585/mmwr.mm6709a4] [PMID: 29518066]

[3]   Islam M, Khatun M, Saha S, Basir M, Hasan M-M. Molecular Detection of *Brucella spp.* from Milk of Seronegative Cows from Some Selected Area in Bangladesh Journal of Pathogens 2018; 2018

[4]   Gul S, Khan A. Epidemiology and epizootiology of brucellosis: A review. Pak Vet J 2007; 27(3): 145.

[5]   Cash-Goldwasser S, Maze MJ, Rubach MP, *et al.* Risk Factors for Human Brucellosis in Northern Tanzania. Am J Trop Med Hyg 2018; 98(2): 598-606.
[http://dx.doi.org/10.4269/ajtmh.17-0125] [PMID: 29231152]

[6]   García Casallas JC, Villalobos Monsalve W, Arias Villate SC, Fino Solano IM. Acute liver failure complication of brucellosis infection: a case report and review of the literature. J Med Case Reports 2018; 12(1): 62.
[http://dx.doi.org/10.1186/s13256-018-1576-4] [PMID: 29519244]

[7]   Matope G, Muma JB, Toft N, *et al.* Evaluation of sensitivity and specificity of RBT, c-ELISA and fluorescence polarisation assay for diagnosis of brucellosis in cattle using latent class analysis. Vet Immunol Immunopathol 2011; 141(1-2): 58-63.
[http://dx.doi.org/10.1016/j.vetimm.2011.02.005] [PMID: 21419497]

[8]   Gupte S, Kaur T. Diagnosis of human brucellosis. Journal of Tropical Diseases & Public Health 2015.

[9]   Meng F, Pan X, Tong W. Rifampicin *versus* streptomycin for brucellosis treatment in humans: A meta-analysis of randomized controlled trials. PLoS One 2018; 13(2)e0191993
[http://dx.doi.org/10.1371/journal.pone.0191993] [PMID: 29462155]

[10]   Majzoobi MM, Hashemi SH, Mamani M, Keramat F, Poorolajal J, Ghasemi Basir HR. Effect of hydroxychloroquine on treatment and recurrence of acute brucellosis: a single-blind, randomized clinical trial. Int J Antimicrob Agents 2018; 51(3): 365-9.
[http://dx.doi.org/10.1016/j.ijantimicag.2017.08.009] [PMID: 28826825]

CHAPTER 39

Trench Fever: A *Bartonella Quintana* Infection

Muhammad Imran Qadir[*] and **Basra Manzoor**

Institute of Molecular Biology & Biotechnology, Bahauddin Zakariya University, Multan, Pakistan

Abstract: Trench fever is an infectious disease for which a specific form of bacteria *Bartonella quintana* is responsible. This infection is characterized by high fever occurring in a single attack or at repeated intervals of 4-5 days, headache, relapses and severe pain in legs and back. It may be diagnosed by culture test, serologic, biopsy, or PCR. Management for this infection is possible in immunologically strong patients by appropriate antibiotics and surgery.

Keywords: *Bartonella quintana*, Doxycycline, Endocarditis, Serologic, Surgery.

INTRODUCTION

Trench fever is an epidemic disease for which the basic reservoir is *Bartonella quintnana*. This infection is also called as 5 days fever. Medical presses of different nations reported a variety of names for trench fever *i.e.* Typhus Mineur and La Fever des Tranches in France, Wolhynian fever in Germany and Gaiter pain fever in Austria. The term trench was given by British forces [1]. Trench fever is an infection transmitted from one person to another person by a body louse containing the responsible agent for it. Bacteria grow in the midgut of lice and transmitted *via* broken skin through crushed lice. Trench fever may be characterized by either a single period of fever or may occur at repeated intervals of 4-5 days.

CAUSES

Initially described etiologic agent for trench fever in 1915 was known as Rickettsia Quintana or *R. Volhynia*. Systematic Bacteriology of Bergey's manual edition 1984 combined all the related forms of this bacteria and after a thorough research Bartonella species were formed [2]. The causative agent for trench fever is a small intracellular, facultative protobacterium *Bartonella quintana* [3].

[*] **Corresponding author Muhammad Imran Qadir:** Institute of Molecular Biology and Biotechnology, Bahauddin Zakariya University, Multan, Pakistan; Tel: +92-61-9210071; Ext. 1920; Fax: +92-61-9210068; E-mail: mrimranqadir@hotmail.com

Muhammad Imran Qadir (Ed.)
All rights reserved-© 2020 Bentham Science Publishers

B quintana infection was excessively observed during World War I in almost every continent except Antarctica and Australia, in those people who suffered from alcoholism, poverty, or homelessness. But most cases were concerned with alcoholism. There is a critical role of body louse for transmission of infection [4].

PREVALENCE

Initially, a term Febris Volhynia was used for trench fever in Poland and followed by the whole of Europe. From Europe the disease transferred to Mesopotamia, Egypt and infections were also observed among those people being in contact with troops returning to England. Trench fever cases also observed in France and Romani [5]. Now the causative agent of this infection is re-appearing in homeless people of Europe being the reason for endocarditis, asymptomatic bacteremia and bacillary angiomatosis [3].

SYMPTOMS

- High-grade fever [6]
- Headache causing pain behind the eyes.
- Conjunctival infection.
- High rate of pain in legs and back.
- A temporary macular or papular rash and sometimes hepatomegaly, splenomegaly are observed.
- Endocarditis may cause complications in some situations.
- Relapses are commonly observed and have continuously occurred to 10 years after primary attack.

DIAGNOSIS

Culture Test

The victim is identified by culture of blood; however, growth may be of 1-4 weeks. The disease is confirmed by persistent bacteremia during a primary attack, relapses throughout the non-symptomatic periods b/w relapses and in victims with endocarditis.

Serologic

Serologic testing is a commonly used method for trench fever diagnosis. Immunofluorescence is used as a reference method [2].

High titration of 1gG antibodies should elucidate endocarditis.

PCR

PCR tests of blood or tissue samples can be performed. Bartonella infections are usually confirmed by taking DNA samples and performing qPCR [7].

Biopsy

Biopsy of skin, valves of heart, lymph nodes, or other tissues [8].

MANAGEMENT

Now antibiotics are recommended for every type of syndrome associated with *B. quintana* in immunologically strong patients.

Medicine

It has been reported that in initial cases of trench fever quinine was used as a drug for treatment. As it was proved effective against malaria having similar symptoms with this fever, it was considered that it would be equally effective against it but it revealed no effect on the natural way of this disease. So other effective drugs were developed against this infectious disease [1].

Doxycycline treatment causes recovery from symptoms in 24-48 hrs. Tetracycline and ceftriaxone (third-generation cephalosporine) are also effective against trench fever. Recovery is mostly complete and mortality is negligible, bacteremia may exist for months after clinical recovery and doxycycline treatment may be required. Patients are given doxycycline 100m e(g/kg/day for 2 weeks of the beginning. Body lice should be controlled. Patients with chronic bacteremia must be monitored for the symptoms of endocarditis. Microbiologic studies accurately predict clinical efficacy as *B. quintana* seems to respond clinically to bacteriostatic agents *i.e.* erythromycin and azithromycin. Only gentamicin is bactericidal *in vitro* because it does not achieve a bactericidal level within human erythrocytes. Gentamicin is not considered to be optimal for monotherapy but it is regularly used in combination with doxycycline [9].

Surgery

Surgical biopsy is possible to manage a proper diagnosis of *B quintana* endocarditis, bacillar angiomatosis or lymphadenitis. In *B quintana* endocarditis situations, valvular heart surgery is required [8].

PREVENTION

- Management of bathing facilities.
- Management of laundry facilities.
- Insecticide application or proper boiling of bedding in shelters.
- Lice affliction treatment by ivermectin.
- Efficient application of infection concerned to *B. quintana* to lower sources of the responsible pathogen [2, 10].

CONSENT FOR PUBLICATION

Not applicable.

CONFLICT OF INTEREST

The authors declare no conflict of interest, financial or otherwise.

ACKNOWLEDGEMENTS

Declared none.

REFERENCES

[1]   Atenstaedt RL. Trench fever: the British medical response in the Great War. J R Soc Med 2006; 99(11): 564-8.
        [http://dx.doi.org/10.1177/014107680609901114] [PMID: 17082300]

[2]   Foucault C, Brouqui P, Raoult D. *Bartonella quintana* characteristics and clinical management. Emerg Infect Dis 2006; 12(2): 217-23.
        [http://dx.doi.org/10.3201/eid1202.050874] [PMID: 16494745]

[3]   Diatta G, Mediannikov O, Sokhna C, *et al.* Prevalence of *Bartonella quintana* in patients with fever and head lice from rural areas of Sine-Saloum, Senegal. Am J Trop Med Hyg 2014; 91(2): 291-3.
        [http://dx.doi.org/10.4269/ajtmh.13-0685] [PMID: 24799368]

[4]   Ohl ME, Spach DH. *Bartonella quintana* and urban trench fever. Clin Infect Dis 2000; 31(1): 131-5.
        [http://dx.doi.org/10.1086/313890] [PMID: 10913410]

[5]   Byam W, Lloyd L. Trench Fever: Its Epidemiology and Endemiology. Proceedings of the Royal Society of Medicine. 1-27.

[6]   Doudier B, Brouqui P. Trench Fever Hunter's Tropical Medicine and Emerging Infectious Disease. 9th ed. Elsevier 2012; pp. 561-3.

[7]   Amanzougaghene N, Fenollar F, Sangaré AK, *et al.* Detection of bacterial pathogens including potential new species in human head lice from Mali. PLoS One 2017; 12(9)e0184621
        [http://dx.doi.org/10.1371/journal.pone.0184621] [PMID: 28931077]

[8]   Raoult D, Fournier P-E, Vandenesch F, *et al.* Outcome and treatment of Bartonella endocarditis. Arch Intern Med 2003; 163(2): 226-30.
        [http://dx.doi.org/10.1001/archinte.163.2.226] [PMID: 12546614]

[9]   Rolain JM, Brouqui P, Koehler JE, Maguina C, Dolan MJ, Raoult D. Recommendations for treatment of human infections caused by Bartonella species. Antimicrob Agents Chemother 2004; 48(6): 1921-33.

[http://dx.doi.org/10.1128/AAC.48.6.1921-1933.2004] [PMID: 15155180]

[10]   Badiaga S, Raoult D, Brouqui P. Preventing and controlling emerging and reemerging transmissible diseases in the homeless. Emerg Infect Dis 2008; 14(9): 1353-9.
[http://dx.doi.org/10.3201/eid1409.080204] [PMID: 18760000]

CHAPTER 40

Urinary Tract Infection: An Infection Caused by Gram-Negative Bacteria especially *E. coli*

Muhammad Imran Qadir[*] and **Muhammad Mubashar Idrees**

Institute of Molecular Biology & Biotechnology, Bahauddin Zakariya University, Multan, Pakistan

Abstract: Urinary Tract Infection (UTI) occurs due to inflammation of the urinary tract including bladder, urethra and kidneys by invading gram-negative bacteria especially *E. coli*. Signs and symptoms of UTI are fever, vomiting, nausea and irritation during urination. Clinical diagnosis is done by using a nitrite test and microbial culture on Cysteine Lactose Electrolyte Deficient (CLED) media plates. Penicillin, cephalosporin, carbapenem and some other antibiotics are used to cure this infection.

Keywords: Gram-Negative Bacteria, Microbial Culture, Urinary Tract Infection.

INTRODUCTION

Urinary tract infection is more prevalent in our community and also leading to death due to its severity. The urinary tract consists of two ureters, a bladder, two kidneys, and urethra. Inflammation in any part of the urinary tract due to the invading of gram-negative bacteria is called urinary tract infection [1].

E. coli enters into the urinary tract system in two ways as an ascending route in which the bacteria move through the urethra into the bladder and then moves into the ureter and kidneys. Another way is called a hematogenous (blood-borne infection) route in which bacteria enter due to inflammation of kidney parenchyma. The risk factor to cause UTI through the hematogenous route has been reduced to a large extent by gram-negative bacteria as compared to the ascending route. *E. coli* is a more common bacteria that cause UTI in both male and female due to invading in the urinary tract [2]. Other bacteria like *Klebsiella spp* and *Proteus spp* are also responsible to cause this infection. *E. coli* usually

[*] **Corresponding author Muhammad Imran Qadir:** Institute of Molecular Biology and Biotechnology, Bahauddin Zakariya University, Multan, Pakistan; Tel: +92-61-9210071; Ext. 1920; Fax: +92-61-9210068; E-mail: mrimranqadir@hotmail.com

Muhammad Imran Qadir (Ed.)
All rights reserved-© 2020 Bentham Science Publishers

present in our body as normal flora in the gastrointestinal tract and also a major part of our microbiome [3]. There are different types of UTI as cystitis (infection in the bladder), urethritis (infection in the urethra), pyelonephritis (infection in the kidney), and prostatitis (prostate infection). Urinary tract inflammation is divided into lower tract inflammation (urethritis, cystitis) and upper tract inflammation (pyelonephritis) Fig. (**13**) [4]. Females have more probability to acquire this infection due to the nearest of urethra and anus and small urethra as compared to males [5, 6].

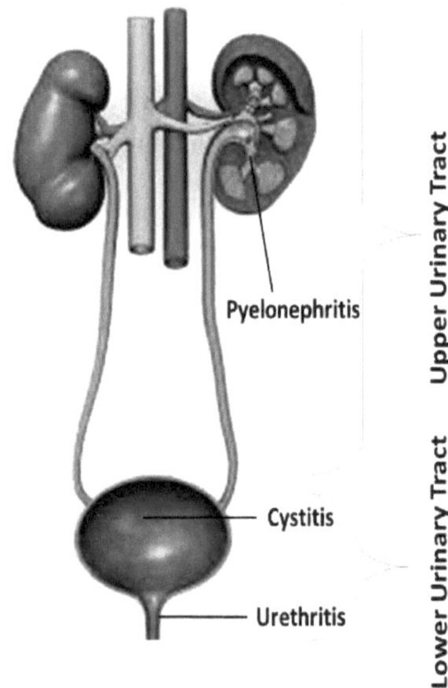

Fig. (13). Sites for urinary tract infection.

SYMPTOMS

Sign and symptom vary from patient to patient due to variation in the site of inflammation and route through which bacteria enter into the urinary tract. Inflammation in different parts results in different symptoms. Fever, dizziness, vomiting and severe pain in the abdomen are observed in kidney disorder [4]. Passing urine continuously with time, blood drainage through urine, and abdomen pain are seen in bladder disorder. Felling discomfort during urination is a major symptom of urethra disorder. Some other symptoms are also observed like urine color is cloudy due to the presence of pus and blood [7]. In the case of asymptomatic bacteriuria, symptoms of UTI are not appeared mostly [8].

DIAGNOSIS

The diagnosis of UTI is done by collecting a urine sample in a sterile urine container. A urine sample is preserved in a refrigerator at 4°C. The sample is preceded within 24 hours otherwise contamination occurs. A nitrite test is performed to check the presence of bacteria in a urine sample. Nitrite test is positive when bacteria are present in urine otherwise negative in the absence of bacteria. After confirmation, the urine sample is inoculated onto the CLED plate by using a disposable plastic wire loop and placed it into the incubator at 37°C for one day. CLED media is used to differentiate between lactose fermenter and non-fermenter. Bacteria grow and pure colonies isolate for the next proceeding [9]. Bacterial colonies are used to perform gram staining for differentiation between gram-positive and negative bacteria. Gram-positive bacteria usually come due to contamination or improper handling of the urine sample. Gram-negative bacteria are used to check which type of bacterial strain cause UTI and performed biochemical test for this purpose. The indole test is used for the detection of *E.coli* which is responsible to cause UTI [10]. *E. coli* shows resistance against antibiotics due to the presence of *bla*$_{CTX-M}$ and *bla*$_{TEM}$ gene [9].

MANAGEMENT

Treatment against UTI is done by using antibiotics against bacteria for two purposes including bactericidal (kill bacteria) and bacteriostatic (stop the multiplication of bacteria). Antibiotics are used to reduce the sign and symptoms of infection. Different types of antibiotics are used according to the sign and symptoms, age, and strain of bacteria causing disease. Mostly nitrofurantoin, fosfomycin, cefotaxime, ceftazidime, ciprofloxacin, cotrimoxazole, levofloxacin, meropenem and imipenem are used [7]. Fluoroquinolones are the choice of drug to cure UTI which is a combination of levofloxacin, ciprofloxacin, and some other antibiotics. These antibiotics are not used in case of mild infection [8]. We should avoid self-medication. Antibiotics are used in the Physician's advice [10].

CONSENT FOR PUBLICATION

Not applicable.

CONFLICT OF INTEREST

The authors declare no conflict of interest, financial or otherwise.

ACKNOWLEDGEMENTS

Declared none.

REFERENCES

[1]   Strouse AC. Appraising the literature on bathing practices and catheter-associated urinary tract infection prevention. Urol Nurs 2015; 35(1): 11-7.
[http://dx.doi.org/10.7257/1053-816X.2015.35.1.11] [PMID: 26298937]

[2]   Flores-Mireles AL, Walker JN, Caparon M, Hultgren SJ. Urinary tract infections: epidemiology, mechanisms of infection and treatment options. Nat Rev Microbiol 2015; 13(5): 269-84.
[http://dx.doi.org/10.1038/nrmicro3432] [PMID: 25853778]

[3]   Abraham SN, Miao Y. The nature of immune responses to urinary tract infections. Nat Rev Immunol 2015; 15(10): 655-63.
[http://dx.doi.org/10.1038/nri3887] [PMID: 26388331]

[4]   Lane DR, Takhar SS. Diagnosis and management of urinary tract infection and pyelonephritis. Emergency medicine clinics 2011; 29(3): 539-2.
[http://dx.doi.org/10.1016/j.emc.2011.04.001]

[5]   Nowicki B. Urinary tract infection in pregnant women: old dogmas and current concepts regarding pathogenesis. Curr Infect Dis Rep 2002; 4(6): 529-35.
[http://dx.doi.org/10.1007/s11908-002-0041-z] [PMID: 12433330]

[6]   Gupta K, Hooton TM, Naber KG, *et al.* International clinical practice guidelines for the treatment of acute uncomplicated cystitis and pyelonephritis in women: A 2010 update by the Infectious Diseases Society of America and the European Society for Microbiology and Infectious Diseases. Clin Infect Dis 2011; 52(5): e103-20.
[http://dx.doi.org/10.1093/cid/ciq257] [PMID: 21292654]

[7]   Salvatore S, Salvatore S, Cattoni E, *et al.* Urinary tract infections in women. Eur J Obstet Gynecol Reprod Biol 2011; 156(2): 131-6.
[http://dx.doi.org/10.1016/j.ejogrb.2011.01.028] [PMID: 21349630]

[8]   Ferroni M, Taylor AK. Asymptomatic bacteriuria in noncatheterized adults. Urol Clin North Am 2015; 42(4): 537-45.
[http://dx.doi.org/10.1016/j.ucl.2015.07.003] [PMID: 26475950]

[9]   Colgan R, Williams M, Johnson JR. Diagnosis and treatment of acute pyelonephritis in women. Am Fam Physician 2011; 84(5): 519-26.
[PMID: 21888302]

[10]   Farrell DJ, Morrissey I, De Rubeis D, Robbins M, Felmingham D. A UK multicentre study of the antimicrobial susceptibility of bacterial pathogens causing urinary tract infection. J Infect 2003; 46(2): 94-100.
[http://dx.doi.org/10.1053/jinf.2002.1091] [PMID: 12634070]

SUBJECT INDEX

A

Abdominal pain fever 47
Abscess 46, 47, 79
  brown 79
Aches, joint 49
Acids 11, 17, 98, 100, 136
  gastric 136
  nucleic 98, 100
  para-aminosalicylic 17
Actinomadura madurae 61
Actinomadura pelletieri 61
Actinomycetes 12, 61
Actinomycetoma 60, 61, 62
Adhesion fimbriae protein 144
Agents 23, 61, 70, 74, 112, 156, 159, 173
  anti-bacterial 61
  antimicrobial 156
  anti-microbial 159
  bacteriostatic 173
  disease-causing 74
  environmental 112
  etiological 61
  immunosuppressive 159
  of nosocomial urinary tract infection 157
  oral 70
  pathogenic 23
Agglutination 23, 24, 96, 125, 126
    reaction 96
    slide TTGA 125
Air 3, 6, 8, 14, 56, 69, 75, 82, 99, 118, 119, 124
  contaminated 124
  impure 99
    passages 6, 8
    pollution 82
    pressure 75
Alectorobius sonrai 50
Allergic reactions 54
Aminoglycosides 153
Amyloidosis 34
Anorexia 58, 167
Anthracis 1, 3, 4
Anthrax 1, 2, 3, 4

cutaneous 1, 2, 4
gastrointestinal 1, 3
inhalational 1, 2, 3, 4
  meningitis 3
Antibacterial 35, 70
  action 35
  activity 70
Antibiotic resistance 69, 71, 72, 88
  in humans and animals 71
Antibiotic(s) 9, 24, 48, 66, 68, 72, 88, 93, 110, 131, 144, 149, 152, 159
  bactericidal 152
  beta-lactam 68
  broad-spectrum 72, 159
  compromised 144
  endogenous 149
  generation 9
  intravenous 134
  macrolide 110
  steroid 131
  tetracycline 93, 144
    therapy 9, 24, 48, 88
    treatment for Bubonic plague 66
Antibodies 24, 56, 57, 65, 93, 100, 115, 120, 125, 130, 131, 134, 140, 141, 145, 148, 168
  detection 93, 168
  monoclonal 65, 125
  oral 131
  pneumoniae 93
Anticonvulsants 115
Antigen detection 93, 110
  sensitive 110
  methods 93
Antigens 3, 17, 23, 24, 49, 65, 96, 109, 141, 161, 162
  cell wall 3
  surface 49
Antigen screening 143, 151
  method 143
Antimicrobial 1, 3, 60, 71, 87
  drugs 1, 3
  susceptibility 87
Anti-tuberculosis drugs 17

Muhammad Imran Qadir (Ed.)
All rights reserved-© 2020 Bentham Science Publishers

Y

Z

www.ingramcontent.com/pod-product-compliance
Lightning Source LLC
Chambersburg PA
CBHW042039110726
48006CB00002B/237